IF I'M NOT HYPOTHYROID, WHAT'S WRONG?

The Multidimensional Approach to Getting Your Energy Back

Audra Whatley, LAc, CFMP

BALBOA.PRESS
A DIVISION OF HAY HOUSE

Balboa Press books may be ordered through booksellers or by contacting:

Balboa Press
A Division of Hay House
1663 Liberty Drive
Bloomington, IN 47403
www.balboapress.com
844-682-1282

Because of the dynamic nature of the Internet, any web addresses or links contained in this book may have changed since publication and may no longer be valid. The views expressed in this work are solely those of the author and do not necessarily reflect the views of the publisher, and the publisher hereby disclaims any responsibility for them.

The author of this book does not dispense medical advice or prescribe the use of any technique as a form of treatment for physical, emotional, or medical problems without the advice of a physician, either directly or indirectly. The intent of the author is only to offer information of a general nature to help you in your quest for emotional and spiritual well-being. In the event you use any of the information in this book for yourself, which is your constitutional right, the author and the publisher assume no responsibility for your actions.

Any people depicted in stock imagery provided by Getty Images are models, and such images are being used for illustrative purposes only. Certain stock imagery © Getty Images.

Print information available on the last page.

ISBN: 978-1-9822-7578-5 (sc)
ISBN: 978-1-9822-7579-2 (e)

Balboa Press rev. date: 10/29/2021

To my overworked, tired, and frustrated patients who just wanted to feel better and, once they did, encouraged me to write this book.

Contents

CHAPTER 1

TIRED, FOGGY, AND FLUFFY

Y GUESS IS, IF YOU PICKED UP THIS BOOK, YOU ARE A smart, savvy individual who is generally in touch with your body and pretty intuitive when something is not quite right. Over the last few years, you've been busy, but you've also noticed things in your body shifting. At first, these changes were subtle – a pound or two here and there, a photograph where your cheeks looked extra puffy, less and less energy to get out and do things. You started to notice the little hair ball in your shower after conditioning your hair was larger than it used to be, and after many weeks of this, you started to wonder if you were going to have any hair left.

Your children are getting older and are in school during the day, but it still doesn't feel like enough of a break to regain your energy and take care of everything you have to do. Dinners become more a task, and you choose easy meals that your family will actually eat instead of healthy ones (if you were ever clear on what you felt "healthy" was in the first place). You may have noticed that you feel lethargic and a little depressed more frequently. Some days, you wish you could just be lazy all day and do absolutely nothing. Although, even when you could indulge in the guilty pleasure of a stay-at-home movie day on the couch, it didn't fix the tiredness.

You feel cold all the time and wear extra layers, even though everyone else wears sleeveless shirts or can leave the house without a jacket during winter. Winter is the worst! Not only are you cold and tired, but your skin is dry and you don't want to leave the house at all. But life calls – your children have to be picked up and taken to various activities.

You may have had a death in the family a while back. You feel like you should be over the grief, but it sneaks back in and the sadness seems to well up over a commercial or something silly while you watch a sitcom. You start to wonder if it will ever get better or if you should be doing something about it; you might even blame it on hormones. You don't want to take antidepressants and have seen counselors in the past, so you know your mind-set is fine – but it still sneaks up on you from time to time.

You've had relationships come and go. Some you look fondly back on, others make you angry. You've had successes and losses in career, family, and life, and you have more responsibility now than you ever imagined you would. Some of these responsibilities you love more than others.

You are getting older, and your hormones are changing. You wonder if this could be part of the problem as well. You write off your irregular menstrual cycles, cramps, PMS, and increased fatigue around your period as a normal part of aging. Or the warm glows in the middle of getting ready for work are just par for the course.

You always feel tired and sometimes foggy-brained, even when you are at a fun family event that you'd usually enjoy. You run around getting selfies and chatting with relatives, only to find yourself looking for the chair at the table in the corner so you can be out of the limelight for a little bit. When you go to bed at night, your mind still twirls around the events of the week and how tired you are, even though your muscles don't feel exhausted or heavy. You fall asleep with one ear awake so you can hear any noises from the kids.

One day, your friend started to talk about how she was feeling the same way you are. She went to her doctor and found out she had hypothyroidism. She was given a prescription and within days, she started to feel better. You googled hypothyroidism later that night and went down the list of symptoms saying, "Yes, yes, yep, that too." You realized you must have hypothyroid as well.

No one wants to be medicated for the rest of their life, but if this was the answer that would get you back to feeling like yourself again, then bring it on. You scheduled your doctor's appointment, went in for labs, and waited for the results.

Finally, your doctor's office called in just to say, "Your labs look fine, other than your cholesterol being a little elevated. Eat right and exercise more."

It's weird to feel disappointed by not getting diagnosed with what you were sure was wrong. However, you don't have hypothyroidism; how could that be? You had every symptom on the checklist. Now what? Maybe you googled some more, tried random supplements, or are just resigned to it being the way it is. The truth is, you feel betrayed by your body. Surely this can't be normal aging?

You were left feeling confused and even frustrated. You wondered, "Did something get missed at the lab? Or is this like taking your car to the shop – it never does that thing when the mechanic drives it." Did your body have one of those days where it was just okay that day?

A year goes by and you are still tired. You have irregular menstrual cycles, your hair is falling out, you have dry skin, you've gained another seven to ten pounds, and having to try on a larger pants' size doesn't make you feel better, by any means. Sure, the pants are more comfortable, but you haven't done anything that would warrant buying larger clothes. You actually have been eating less and better, but you are too tired to care anymore. You just buy larger pants anyway, because you have to have clothes to wear that don't feel like they are cutting you in half.

You go back to your doctor and tell the same story again. "I'm still tired, in a bit of a funk. My weight went up, as your nurse noted when she took it. Something has to be wrong."

The doctor says, "Well, your labs still look fine … do I need to put you on a statin or are you going to try to eat better this year? If your mood is your primary concern, I can prescribe an antidepressant." You refuse the antidepressant because being in a funk isn't depressed! And if you weren't so disappointed that your thyroid still showed up as normal, you might want to jab his eyes out for the "eat better this year" comment, but it didn't even occur to you until hours later.

How long is this going to go on until you find answers and got some help from someone? You read about foods to support you online. One page says eat plenty of vegetables and the next says broccoli and kale are bad for your thyroid. The following site says take iodine and the following one says that it could trigger autoimmune issues. The information is as confusing as the symptoms themselves. You are ready to pull your hair out, but it's clear you don't need to because it is already thinner, finer, and less shiny than ever; it's already falling out on its own.

Now what? Should you look for alternatives? Should you see an acupuncturist, naturopath or holistic doctor of some sort? Who do you go to? Would that be weird or a waste of time and money? Those are both already concerns. You make it by okay and have a nice place to live, but you still worry about college funds, updating cars, and something breaking on the house. Can you afford to spend money on something you can't even prove you have?

You opt to try one of those supplements at the health food store. After all, it says it improves metabolism, helps with weight loss, and boosts energy. But you followed the directions and noticed nothing. Your computer pops up an ad on your email about why your thyroid isn't working. You watch the video; it seems to tell your story and offers a special for supplements that are doctor-recommended. The supplements are supposed to be more effective than anything out there. So, you try that too, and it doesn't work either.

At this point, you are ready to throw in the towel on supplements, diets, and doctors, but that would also mean throwing in the towel on your own health. You can't do that, for the sake of your children, spouse, and future. You just want to understand what the problem is and start to feel like yourself again.

You think surely there is someone out there who has been through this and found answers! Someone who overcame the fatigue and stopped losing all her hair. Someone who would be willing to help you find out what's actually going on and what to do about it. There is! Let me tell you my story.

CHAPTER 2

JOURNEY OF WELL-BEING

FROM A YOUNG AGE, I KNEW THAT I WANTED TO WORK AT THE deepest levels of healing, assisting those around me. As far as my public school–taught, logical yet naïve sixteen-year-old brain could understand, the best way to do that was at the genetic level. I found the only school in Texas that had a genetics program in the early 1990s – Texas A&M University. While I would have preferred human studies, the Agricultural and Life Sciences school there led the way and was known globally for their genomic research. I had always considered myself healthy, other than the occasional cold or sinus infection and the common seasonal allergies that everyone in the piney woods of Southeast Texas seemed to have.

Throughout my undergraduate career, as I learned more about evolutionary biology and genetic diseases, two things became clear to me. First, I realized every bit of our bodies – genetic material, hair, eyeballs and insides – are just made of carbon, hydrogen, oxygen, and a little nitrogen and other elements. All of those, at their core, were only positive, negative, and neutral particles, but particles of what? I wasn't sure and didn't give it that much thought at the time. All I knew was this was our deepest understood level of biology.

The second thing that became clear was that of a group of one hundred people with the same gene for whatever disease, there was "varying expressivity or a lack of penetrance," meaning that some people with the disease show symptoms, and some don't. Whether they do or do not isn't related to their genetics, but more so to their environment and what seemed like mysterious luck. These two ideas seemed to be the same questions that were pondered by the PhDs in the graduate lab that I worked in, but no one had any answers and were primarily involved in finding answers to their own research projects. I let it go for the time being.

After graduation, I worked with several research teams. I helped create diagnostic testing for bone marrow matching and identifying wildlife populations with prion disease (this was the decade of mad cow disease research) and then created vaccines for companion animals for a veterinary science company. During this time, I had a lingering sinus infection that I just could not seem to shake. Round after round of antibiotics seemed to help for a week or so, but then it would come back. My health spiraled into breathing treatments, inhalers, and managing asthma that I didn't have before this experience.

After eighteen months of misery, and while debating going to med school and studying for the MCATs, I asked for advice at an organic food market supplement section. The young man working there replied with certainty, "Dude, why don't you try these herbs!" At the time, I was desperate for relief, so I did. Three days later, the congestion, difficulty breathing, and asthma went away and stayed away for nearly six months. When the symptoms came back, I went and bought the herbs again and had similar results.

It was at this moment that my mind was made up – I wanted to look for a medical system based in herbs, which is how I found Traditional Chinese Medicine (TCM). As far as my limited research could tell, it was the most intricate and complete program for herbology available. When I enrolled in acupuncture school, I had never actually had acupuncture; in fact, I had a healthy fear of needles. But, the program blew my mind at how well it tied together so many of the experiences I watched family members go through with their health. It gave me a well-rounded picture that my science background seemed to have missed in its compartmentalized-systems approach.

To say the least, I fell in love with TCM. But I also came to realize its shortcomings. I wanted the same things I did when I entered the science field – answers to how to fix health problems for good, not just treat the symptoms. Herbs often worked to relieve symptoms, but when you stopped them, much like medications, the symptoms could come back. Mind you, Chinese medicine was a much gentler approach that, with a little diligence, made a huge difference in overcoming many of the health challenges that the medicine I had seen and experienced had not, but it still didn't have all of the answers I wanted especially for chronic, long term health concerns.

During my acupuncture/graduate school days, I started feeling fatigued and gaining more weight than I would have liked. At my yearly doctor's visit, I was told that I was fine; I was just getting older and needed to eat right and exercise more. "Just getting older?" I thought. I was still in my mid-twenties! That was definitely not what I wanted to hear.

Over the next five years, I tried several diets, where I would lose a little weight, gain a little more back, and start over again with the next best diet I could find. It seemed unfair and frustrating beyond belief that the people around me doing the same programs lost significantly more weight and were able to keep it off. I was tired more often, which made the trips to the gym seem like a daunting task, but I went anyway. On the days I didn't have early classes, I slept in. I had always been a night owl who didn't like to get up early, but on the days I slept nine to ten hours and still felt tired, I had to wonder what was wrong with me. It didn't seem normal or healthy.

After graduating with Masters of Science in Oriental Medicine, I moved back up to my favorite Front Range location in

Colorado and started my practice. Three months later, my father passed away. Between the sadness and grief of losing my father and of miserably failing at my first attempt in business, I moved back to Texas. I was closer to family, and the economy and cost of living seemed to be easier, allowing me to start over. All this time, my weight increased, and my energy decreased, but I just kept going. My doctors continued to say I was fine, repeating that my cholesterol was a little high, but if I ate right and exercised, everything would be normal.

I threw myself into working out every day – sometimes twice, if I knew the personal trainer would be there. One thing my trainer stressed was that you can't outrun, out-workout, or outsmart a bad diet. So, I tried my best to eat healthier, according to what the doctor told me; I consumed less fat (margarine instead of butter), egg whites for protein, carbohydrates for fuel, and plenty of low-fat dairy for calcium and vitamin D, with vegetables too, of course. I know some of you just rolled your eyes at this "heart healthy" diet from the 1980s, but it was still recommended at the time. Admittedly, I got closer to the weight I had been when I graduated college, I had more energy, but I still did not feel 100 percent and struggled to keep up the pace I set for myself.

At the ripe old age of thirty, I hurt my back lifting more weight than I should have. Working out became a thing of the past and regular chiropractic visits kept me walking without pain shooting down my legs for the next few months. Jogging would flare up my pain, as did jumping, dancing, and boot camp classes. I tried yoga, and while definitely not my thing, it did seem to help my back. Additionally, yoga was something I could squeeze in between starting a practice, waiting tables, and teaching night classes at the massage school.

To say the least, I was tired, and on the weekends, I slept as much as possible or was a couch potato for as long as I could be. Relationships came and went; my practice began to gain momentum, and I was able to let go of the extra jobs. My weight jumped up ten pounds in a week or two and then stabilized, even though I hadn't changed anything. I ate less and tried to exercise more, but had little success.

A friend suggested that I might have hypothyroid issues, so I looked it up on the internet. I read through the symptom list, thinking, "Fatigue? Yep, too often. Weakness? I definitely can't maintain exercise or lift heavy weight anymore; I can't even open the salsa jar. Weight gain, yes, that was a major complaint. Dry skin? Hmm, I thought I just hadn't recovered from the dry mountain climate. Hair loss – *oh my gosh*, my long, shiny hair had become duller and thinner over the last few years. I was also cold more often than ever before. Muscle cramps and achiness? I thought I was just tired, but okay, I have this too. Constipation? I often had that, so I never considered it a symptom. Depression? As much as I don't want to admit it, I've struggled with it off and on for years. Irritability? Yes, especially certain times of the month or when I am around too many people too often. Memory loss – do you mean going to the fridge, opening it, and staring blankly, or going to change the laundry from washer to dryer and realizing several hours later I hadn't made it there? Yep. Abnormal menstrual cycles – you mean my thirty-two- to thirty-five-day, energy-draining, crampy nightmares? Oh yes, that one too. Decreased libido – I hadn't noticed, but my ex would say absolutely yes. Hmmm, maybe my friend was right, I have an answer for my issues!"

I went to my annual doctor's visit, suggested my findings, and she ran a TSH (thyroid-stimulating hormone) test and said, "You're fine. It's not your thyroid. You are just getting older and have been under a lot of stress. I can prescribe an antidepressant to help with that low-grade depression." I was disappointed and refused the antidepressant for reasons that are, as they say in Texas, "a whole 'nother story."

I didn't know what to do at that point, other than just keep going. I picked up a holistic magazine for our area and when I perused through it, I saw an ad for an MD who had gone holistic. She mentioned many of the symptoms I had and natural solutions to them, so I went to check her out. She was adamant that everything going on was because of candida, so she had me do a candida cleanse and take a whole bunch of supplements (some of which made me throw up every night I took them). I tried explaining that to her, and she said it was just the die-off of the candida (like literally dead yeast inside of me – yuck) and told me to keep going and that I would feel better. I tried and kept throwing up every time I took it. After a couple more visits that did not improve my health, ending in my frustration, I quit going to her.

Next, I found a naturopathic doctor to try out, and we did numerous tests and took homeopathic drops; she suggested that I was allergic to a laundry list of foods that I would have to cut out of my diet. As I sat down at lunch later, I cried because there wasn't a single thing on that delicious-looking menu that I could eat, according to her list. I finally settled on a salad, minus the cheese, croutons, dressing, carrots, and tomatoes – I mean, I had a bowl of dry lettuce. I cried some more and left hungry. After about a week of that diet, I did feel better, but also felt like I was starving and knew I couldn't keep it up forever. The homeopath gently and kindly suggested that I hadn't been following the diet as well as expected when my weight had not decreased, but again I did feel somewhat better. However, it didn't take long before I gave up on that too.

A year or so later, another friend recommended her MD, who specialized in unusual thyroid cases. By this time, my face was puffy, I was heavier than I had ever been, the outer thirds of my eyebrows had thinned to almost nothing, and my neck had gotten thick. After much deliberation, I gave my friend's doctor a call and got on her schedule. She said my labs were in normal range, but that I had an obvious goiter, or enlarged thyroid, and she was going to prescribe a compounded natural thyroid medication.

The first couple of days after the medication, I felt amazing for the first time that I could remember. But, that feeling soon faded. So, when I went for my check-up the next month, my doctor upped my dosage. I felt good again, and then I didn't. This went on for months, until my doctor was unwilling to up the dosage anymore. At that point, my brain seemed to be back online. I could think again. My weight wasn't coming down, but I didn't seem to care as much because I felt like moving again and started a boot camp class. I would love to say that I lost the weight and that's the end of my story, but it's not even close.

I wasn't cold all the time, but my face would be beet-red and I felt sweaty with little exertion or if the room was over seventy-four degrees. I often felt anxious and jittery but had no idea why. When my doctor checked my extended hands to see if they had tremors, they did not, so she left me at that dosage. Again, I felt better; I just had a few other things that I learned to manage with more air conditioning, less clothing in the summer, and with learning meditation to calm my emotional reaction to my jittery insides. I was good – sort of.

Later that year, I went on a seventeen-day spiritual journey to Bali. It would be awesome if I could say I had a miraculous spontaneous healing, but I didn't. I did, however, forget to pack my thyroid medication and had no idea how to replace it once I realized it wasn't in my bag. Fortunately for me, I did not end up in a coma from going with out (which I found out later is a potential outcome of going cold turkey off higher dosages of thyroid meds, so *do not do that!*) I spent the majority of my trip in a foggy haze, sleeping through all of the meditations and bus rides, only awake enough to move and take a few pictures when nudged by our leader to do so. I felt like an infant waking only to eat, poop, and smile long enough to convince the others I was okay. Once I returned home, I convinced myself that I had already come through the worst of it, so I would just see how I did without going back on the medication. I felt good for a while.

Six months later, my symptoms began to return. I went back to my thyroid doctor and was put back on increasing dosages of meds, but we stopped at a lesser dosage than before. Soon after, my doctor told me she was retiring and my case would be turned over to someone else. My insurance carrier also changed around the same time and their practice was no longer covered. My insurance company recommended a physician close to my home, and I went in to establish myself there and get a refill on my prescription. This new doctor said she didn't believe in what I was taking and prescribed the standard of care, Synthroid (levothyroxine), at what should have been a similar dosage. I wasn't happy, so I tried to argue for the same prescription I had but was told no. I didn't know what else to do but take it.

A week after being on this new prescription, my allergies started flaring up in ways they hadn't in over a decade. I called my doctor's office to request being put back on the natural thyroid product and was told that it was all in my head; the medication could not cause allergies. I knew beyond a shadow of a doubt it was the only thing that had changed.

As a healthcare provider, I don't recommend what I did next for anyone! However, remember the bottle of compounded thyroid meds I forgot when I went to Bali the year before? That medication was still in my cabinet. I began weaning myself off with that and using essential oils, supplements, and herbs I researched. In a matter of days, my nose cleared, my eyes stopped itching, and my breathing went back to normal. Plus, I didn't feel any different at this point than I did on the original thyroid medication.

In the years that followed my experience, I found other practitioners who had some variation of similar struggles with our medical system and turned to the evidence-based research mentioned in functional medicine instead of the standard of care that was offered. I completed a postgraduate certification in functional medicine in 2016, so I could continue to help myself and others find a better way to relieve their symptoms before they went through what I did.

While I still see acupuncture patients for all sorts of things, I also use functional medicine and laboratory testing to guide my patients to better health. I have come to see that both Eastern philosophy and practices and Western science each has a place and balance each other perfectly. By following what I set out here in the rest of this book, I feel healthier and more alive in my midforties than I ever did in my thirties. My eyebrows returned, and my hair got shiny and grew back in. While I'm not at my perfect weight, I am significantly lighter and clearer-minded and am no longer sensitive to temperature changes, and I have answers that I never even imagined asking the questions to.

As I started putting what I had learned in practice for others, it became clear that not everyone had the same problem even if their symptoms were similar. It would sometimes take using one protocol, then another to get them feeling better and then even better. It was this journey with my patients and the feedback that I received from them helped me understand how to help others even more. They kept saying to me, "I wish I had a book to read about what you are telling me – it's fascinating and makes so much sense for why I am the way I am." Healing on all levels is a journey. Instead of sending you to multiple documentaries, doctors, places, books and modalities, I've taken it all in, let go of what didn't work for me, and put the rest of what is useful all together in one place. It is completely possible you could find your answers on the pages of this book and be able to move forward on your own.

I pray that you haven't been through, and never have to go through, the gamut that I did. My hope is that by reading this book, you can find answers that are healthy and sustainable for you. The biggest question is: Are you ready?

CHAPTER 3

OPEN TO RECEIVING

I T TOOK YEARS FOR ME TO DECIDE TO ACTUALLY WRITE ABOUT my experiences, and many more years to actually get past asking myself, "Who am I to write a book of any sort, much less one talking about health and wellness when I struggled and made mistakes and am still nowhere near the cute, little yoga fitness gurus of the social media world?" When I got past all my insecurities, it occurred to me that no – I am the small-town Texas girl who was "too smart for her own good" and had put together seemingly opposing fields of medicine to make my own way and help those around me in whatever way I could.

I remember one of the doctors I interned under in Chinese medical school telling me, "Put all of that scientific knowledge in a box on a shelf in your mind, and when you have immersed yourself in the philosophy here enough to really understand it, pull out the old shoebox, and put them together." This is what I have done and will continue to do throughout the rest of this book and in practice.

That being said, in the chapters that follow, I will speak science. Hopefully, I will do so in a way that piques your interest, does justice to the science itself, and gives you answers about what is going on in your body from a physiological perspective. I will also give you a glimpse into traditional Chinese medicine and philosophy used by many acupuncturists to diagnose and treat what seems to be unseen in the medical profession. We'll also discuss what it is to be a quantum integrative physician by combining the two and using quantum physics to bridge the gap between the mysterious world of Chinese medicine and the more traditional protocols used here in the United States.

Being an acupuncturist for nearly twenty years, I have heard it all from potential patients who were afraid to experience something different. I calmed people with needle phobias (like myself), turned the skeptics into believers, and helped the fearful understand that Chinese medicine is written in an ancient language that makes it sound different. But Chinese medicine is not all that far off of what you already know from nature when you understand the analogies that it is written in.

Since traditional Chinese medicine is based on an ancient philosophy that was written in analogies of the time, it is often misunderstood or translated in a way that intuitively makes no sense. The Chinese language itself is a bit of a mystery to most of us Westerners, as letters are not used to form words like in English. Instead, Chinese uses a combination of symbols to represent words. The actual symbol for an herb may literally be the symbols for cow and knee, when it is actually a root that looks like a little white stick with knobby middle that looks like a cow knee; more importantly, it is effective with knee and back pain. The other fascinating part about this language is that English has one word for "love," and we use descriptive terms if we want to clarify what it means to us in a particular situation. In Chinese, there are many characters that represent different kinds of love. The opposite is true with more tangible things, such as tree bark, orange peel, skin, and animal hide; there is only one symbol and Chinese uses descriptive symbols to clarify.

I am aware that I am not, and will likely never be, fluent in Chinese. My fascination with the medicine and the language has gotten me to a place where I recognize some of the symbols and can speak a few basic sentences. It's a bit like they teach first and second graders other languages, with basics such as numbers going up to ten, "Hello, how are you," "thank you," and "my name is Audra." Beyond that, I immersed myself in the philosophy, as it was taught in school and in the books that I read after and realized how the philosophy pointed toward spiritual teachings but didn't include them for the purposes of medical education.

The rest of this book is not just traditional Chinese medicine but a dive into the basics of it. The layout has influences of eastern philosophy, but not the traditional teachings. Instead, this book is a culmination of personal growth and development courses, what I learned from spiritual practices, how I interpret the original teachings, and how that can be related to potential thyroid issues.

In Chapter 4, you will learn why your doctor says you are fine and why you are still feeling symptoms that they seem to be ignoring. You will start to learn what has been going on in your body. Chapter 5 starts your journey in Chinese medicine and in your body on the molecular level. We will also tiptoe into quantum physics as it relates to Chinese medicine. In Chapter 6, we then balance physical medicine and Chinese medicine with the theories of quantum physics. I promise it is much easier to understand than it sounds. At this point, I would take a break – notice these principles in your life. Journal about how your outlook is different now and what you have or will discover by starting this journey.

Chapters 7 through 11 look at the five elements individually and walk you through a process of healing. I recommend dedicating at least a week to each chapter and putting the suggestions from each into your life in order and allowing them to build on each other. You may feel uncomfortable in one chapter more than the others – stay there longer. It is natural for us to try to avoid that which is uncomfortable, but that is exactly where your body is screaming for you to spend some more time doing the work. Journal your initial thoughts, your feelings throughout the process and what happens each week or two that relates to that element.

If you put the book down and don't go any further, you are likely stuck in that area and not ready to move on. That is okay, but I suggest picking it up and reading forward.

In my group programs I often spend up to three weeks in the processes of Chapter 7 alone, not talking about what is written, but putting into action the detox and growth processes. While I incorporate some elements of Chapter 8 with my clients from week two to completion of our twelve-week program, I don't actually talk about Chapter 8 until week five.

Chapter 12 links together all five elements in a way that brings more insight and clarity into what has been going on in your body and how to continue to get and stay healthy. Chapter 13 and Chapter 14 tie it all up in a nice little bow and tell you how to find me and my clinic if you want more support in the process. While it is completely doable to read this book cover to cover in a few hours, that in itself is not going to help you feel better. It is taking action or getting support in taking those actions that makes all the difference.

That being said, I invite you to be open to receive. Open your mind to something new, whether it be a scientific explanation, a different way of thinking, or just learning in general. If you need to put some things in a shoebox on a shelf for a bit to do so, then by all means, visualize that shoebox, stuff it full, and wrap it up with some duct tape if it keeps spilling over and clouding your willingness to be present as you read forward.

CHAPTER 4

WHY YOUR DOCTOR
SAYS YOU'RE FINE

No one just wakes up one day with a laundry basket full of hypothyroid symptoms; it is a process that happens over time. Any sort of discomfort in the body, unless it was caused by trauma or infection, doesn't happen overnight. Instead, it is a process of dysfunction over time. When we take a step back and look at the full life cycle of a human being, we get a different perspective than the definition of disease that is used in medicine:

> *"Disease, any harmful deviation from the normal structural or functional state of an organism, generally associated with certain signs and symptoms and differing in nature from physical injury. Thus, the normal condition of an organism must be understood in order to recognize the hallmarks of disease."*
> — The Britannica Dictionary

Later in this chapter, I will refer back to this definition, but for now, let's go back to hypothyroid.

Ideally, we come into this life perfect with optimal health. As we get exposed to environmental threats, our bodies become stressed. We are designed to respond to stress by clearing the offending stressor, moving away from it, or fighting the threat quickly and then returning to normal to rest, digest, ease, and function optimally.

This was the case with our ancient ancestors when they had an adrenaline surge in order to run from a tiger. But then, once safe, their adrenaline levels returned to normal. This is also the case with the infant who cries for their mom – the mom would hear and then take care of whatever threatened the infant's comfort. This is a function of the HPA axis (hypothalamus-pituitary-adrenal), which I will address more in Chapter 11. The short version is that when the brain senses a threat, the hypothalamus sends a message to the pituitary gland that in turn sends a biochemical message to the adrenal glands to release adrenaline. Once the threat is no longer present, the adrenaline in the system acts as a messenger to the hypothalamus to tell the pituitary to send a calming biochemical message to the adrenal glands to release noradrenaline, which neutralizes the adrenaline.

With the advances in our world over the last couple of hundred years, our pace of living has exponentially increased. Our DNA, however, has not evolved much from the time of caveman over 40,000 years ago. So, flying down the highway at eighty miles an hour with cars on either side that could take you out and then quickly braking when someone cuts you off is as stressful to your body as being stalked by a pack of hyenas. While we may be somewhat comfortable at that pace, our HPA axis does not differentiate the threat of a car accident from the threat of a tiger or hyena.

Yet we are accustomed to these threats and many of us feel threatened multiple times a day – before we get to our job, we stress about deadlines and demanding coworker(s), and then we rush to get our children to their extracurricular activities and then inhale a quick lunch while typing away at our computers to meet the aforementioned deadlines so we can avoid a confrontation with the boss who may or may not be looking over our shoulders. This often seems to be the new normal for humans, not to mention the constant bombardment of stressful information from news, commercials, TV shows, and social media. These situations are nothing like the experiences the hunter/gatherers we descended from lived through. Not that I would want to give up my modern comforts for a cave floor, but the pace we live at is exponentially busier and faster than that of one hundred, or even fifty years ago. Wouldn't it be nice to not stress and enjoy a sunset or a leisurely stroll and conversation with a loved one?

After many stressors over and over, day in and day out, our system adapts to its pace and environment as best as it can. Over time, this adaptation wears down our system, as stressors continue coming through an already adapted system. At some point, we become fatigued. Think of the caveman with a broken leg that wasn't set quite right. It heals, he adapts, and can still do his best to escape the tiger. However, he is likely going to be slower than others who are not adapted to a broken limb, so he has to think faster and potentially work harder to avoid being eaten.

One of the first signs people associate with hypothyroid is being tired often and gaining weight. There are many reasons for fatigue, but a stressed body, adapted to manage continued stressors, can only last so long before experiencing fatigue. If your body doesn't get the chance to rest and digest, it just keeps going and creates a sluggish system that is more focused on managing the outside world than dealing with whatever food you managed to eat. In a perfect world, we would leave those stressors at the office and go home to a nice, relaxing environment and a healthy meal, leading to joyful interactions with our loved ones and an early bedtime.

However, that is not reality. Many of us run to get the things done that we couldn't while working, squeeze food in before the next event, or get the kids in bed at a decent hour so that we have an hour or two to do the rest of our chores, like cleaning the kitchen, finishing laundry, and checking emails that popped up since we left work. Eventually, we get to bed with our minds still racing after turning off the TV, phone, and tablet in time to wake up and do it all over again.

Continuing this pattern day in and day out eventually leads to functional abnormalities that you notice but are still considered "normal" and "functional" to the medical community. This is not your doctor's fault. The lab ranges given to your doctor are based on the 5 to 10 percent extremes on each end of a bell curve. Notice the definition of disease from the beginning of this chapter; it is a "harmful deviation from the functional state" that doctors look for. You are still functional, and oftentimes this is considered "normal aging process."

Years may go by in this "functional state" before the symptoms become diagnosable as a physiological condition, such as hypothyroidism or another disease. It is here, at the physiological stage, that our medical system begins to kick in and recognize the dysfunction enough to medicate or take surgical action. The next step after physiological impairment is death. The process of life to death goes like this: optimal, stressed, adapted, fatigued, functional, physiological, death. Medicine and surgery work their best in and between the physiological and death stages.

I want to be clear that I am not against MDs or medicine. Our medical system has some of the best technology in the world for bringing people back to life from the brinks of death and helping get them to a physiological stability. However, medical schools do not teach MDs what, if anything, can be done before people get to this stage of disease process. Assisting people with issues before that stage is not considered medically necessary by the insurance companies and therefore is not covered. The medical system is designed with the problems of the 1910s (Legionnaires' disease), 1920s (plague), 1930s (smallpox), and 1940s and 1950s (polio) in mind, when "find the pathogen and how to kill it" was the forefront of science.

This mind-set somewhat works with diseases that have progressed unnoticed to the physiological stage, like cancer, but does not and cannot be applied to the autoimmune systems or dysfunctions of the metabolic system without killing the individual. The growing numbers of autoimmune and chronic diseases (hypothyroidism falls into this category) is still a bit of a mystery to the medical community. In a recent poll, more than 50 percent of MDs responded that they did not feel comfortable or equipped to diagnose and treat autoimmune or associated diseases. This is where functional medicine, nutrition, and complementary and alternative medicine excel, when given a chance.

The Thyroid: Function and Diagnosis

The standard of care for diagnosing hypothyroid is elevated TSH (thyroid-stimulating hormone) and sometimes low thyroxine (T4). Many MDs are only looking at TSH, which is produced by the pituitary gland in the brain, as the basis for hypothyroidism. TSH is a bit like the parent who knocks on their kids' door saying get up and get to work(or school); TSH becomes louder and more frequent when the kid doesn't seem to be up and going.

Doctors are not looking at how much of the thyroid hormone your body currently produces or converts to usable form. There are two thyroid hormones – the first is thyroxine (T4), which is produced by the thyroid itself. It is a conglomeration of four iodine molecules and tyrosine (an amino acid). T4 must be converted to T3 before it is usable in the body. Triiodothyronine (T3) is the active form of T4 that can be utilized by the body, and is made when one of the iodine molecules of T4 is cleaved off. This process mostly happens in the liver but can also happen in the heart, muscle, gut, and nerves.

Triiodothyronine (T3) helps maintain muscle control, brain function and development, and heart and digestive functions. It also plays a role in the body's metabolic rate and the maintenance of bone health. Thyroxine (T4) primarily acts as a precursor for T3 and is a primary indicator in the feedback loop to the brain to regulate thyroid production. When T4 is elevated, the hypothalamus sends a message to the pituitary to stop sending TSH to the thyroid. When T3 is low, hypothyroid symptoms start to occur. Ideally, T4 properly indicates T3 amounts to the brain. However, my undiagnosed patients often feel all the symptoms of hypothyroid and their TSH and T4 levels are normal, but they are not converting T4 to T3 as efficiently or properly as is required by their body.

You can think of your thyroid symptoms like the smoke alarm in your house. The sound is annoying and only happens for one of two reasons: the battery is low, so it chirps every so often to warn us to give it more energy/fuel (battery), or it plays a loud blaring sound when it detects smoke from a fire somewhere else in the house. The smoke alarm itself is not the problem, only the warning system. If you're like me, to stop the chirping at 3:00 a.m., because the battery always seems to go out in the middle of the night, you use a broom handle to pop out the battery, just to get it to shut up so you can go back to sleep. This fixes the immediate annoyance but does nothing about the low battery it's trying to warn you about and if there is a fire, no alarm will sound. Throughout the rest of this book, you will get a roadmap of what to do about your symptoms, instead of just popping out the battery and ignoring them.

Most people don't even consider seeing a doctor until they have a nagging symptom, or multiple nagging symptoms that can no longer be ignored — in other words, their smoke alarm is blaring. By this point, you are far past discomfort and into full-on misery. Consider yourself wise for making an effort to find answers for the symptoms you experience before they are considered "medically necessary" to treat.

What you've learned so far is that your smoke alarm is chirping at you. It may be useful to look at labs, such as TSH, Free T4, Free T3, Total T4, Reverse T3 and T3 uptake, as well as Thyroglobulin Antibody + Thyroid Peroxidase (TPO) Antibody. These will give you a better picture of what is actually going on. They can be run through your practitioner or services like anylabtestnow.com (which is pricier, but cuts out the doctor fees if you want to do it for yourself.) The two antibodies tell you if your body is creating an autoimmune response, which is what is seen in Hashimoto's disease, while the others just paint a picture of whether or not you are producing and converting thyroid hormones. Notice if the numbers are closer to the upper and lower ends of the "normal" ranges, as these ranges are broader than where symptoms start to occur.

You also learned that our smoke alarm wouldn't be chirping at us if there wasn't something triggering it to do so. Labs only help point us in the direction of what supplements may be useful. The rest of this book dives deeper than the physical and tells you how to help yourself with your symptoms, whether you have the actual test results or not.

CHAPTER 5

YOU ARE MORE
THAN A BODY

THE EMPEROR LOOKED OUT OVER HIS PEOPLE AND SAID TO HIS magistrate, "These modern medicines are killing our people. Go to the royal families and catalog and categorize the medicine used to keep them healthy and vibrant. I want it understandable so that for eons to come it can be passed down." This is a simplified version of the original story told in the *Lingshu* or, *The Spiritual Pivot,* translated by Wu Jing-Nuan about the Yellow Emperor of China who lived and ruled somewhere between 475 and 221 BC. The problems of that time are still relevant today, and this is the reason I include the teachings here. At the foundation of Chinese medicine is the concept of Qi, which we will be talking about throughout this book.

In *The Web That Has No Weaver,* Ted Kaptchuk referred to Qi as follows: "The idea of Qi is fundamental to Chinese medical thinking, yet no one English word or phrase can adequately capture its meaning. We can say that everything in the universe, organic and inorganic, is composed of and defined by its Qi. But Qi is not some primordial, immutable material, nor is it merely vital energy, although the word is occasionally so translated. Chinese thought does not distinguish between matter and energy, but we can perhaps think of Qi as matter on the verge of becoming energy or energy at the point of materializing. Neither the classical nor modern Chinese texts speculate on the nature of Qi, nor do they attempt to conceptualize it. Rather, Qi is perceived by functionally – what it does."

This is where my movie- and comic book–loving, yet scientific mind says, "Wait a minute … that sounds familiar." Energy at the point of becoming matter, matter at the point of becoming energy — isn't that really similar to wave particle theory? Now, I know some of you have no idea what I'm referring to and others just had a lightbulb go off, so let me explain.

In quantum physics, there is something called the "double slit experiment," where electrons are fired at an object with two cut-out slits. Imagine a target board with two cut out rectangles and a screen or canvas behind the target board. In the world of physics, we would expect that shooting at a target like this would leave a pattern on the canvas consistent with firing paint balls at board with those cut outs. However, that is not what happened. When electrons were fired at the target, the pattern that emerged was similar to the pattern produced by light being shined at similar target; light is made of waves.

How did this happen? When an observer was introduced to the experiment, the original expected pattern appeared. After many repeats of this same phenomenon, it became evident that electrons show both properties of matter and wave energy. This is how wave particle theory came to be. Electrons, it turns out, are not the only particles to do this. The same is also true for neutrons, positrons, compound particles like atoms, and even molecules that contain more than one atom. The first time I heard this, my mind was blown. It took several times watching the video for the meaning to even start to sink. If you are a visual person, check out the YouTube video from the movie *What the Bleep* here that explains it: https://www.youtube.com/watch?v=Q1YqgPAtzho.

So, what does this have to do with Qi? Well, as Ted Kaptchuk stated in 1983, no one can ever speculate on the nature of Qi. So, here I am, speculating that somehow thousands of years ago, the ancient Chinese somehow understood the concept that we are made of energy – not the "woo-woo," weird, mystical, fairy world, magical energy, but the scientific, electron-whirling, biochemical energy, down to the smallest particles of our physical body. And it may seem like magic to speak of shifting someone's well-being by expecting it to move in a healthier direction.

Between quantum physics and Chinese medicine, we can start to imagine that if an observer of the wave makes it a particle because that is what is expected, then wouldn't an observer of stagnant matter, who expected it to move as a wave, also be able to make that happen? To take it a step further, the things we already experience as a wave, like emotions, could also be stuck or moving, depending on how we observe them. The traditional Chinese medicine system takes this into account by not only speaking of the physical properties of the body but also about the emotions associated with it.

Now, some of you may wonder what this has to do with your thyroid symptoms. Those symptoms don't come about without some dysfunction somewhere in the body that directly correlates with the putting together and taking apart of molecules. It could be a physical issue, like not having the correct components (atoms) needed to produce thyroid hormones and metabolize them into usable forms, or it could be that something somewhere in the process is stuck from waves of emotion that were stuffed down and never observed again. Or it could be even more than that.

The notion of wave particle theory is often referred to in terms of duality, meaning it has a dual nature – either this or that. Well, human beings also have that dual nature. We are physical bodies that are highly sophisticated and masterful at pulling off trillions of physiological processes in a day without a single conscious thought required.

We are also energetically sensitive, spiritual beings who can be hurt by words, feel slighted by inaction, and put all sorts of meaning to things that may or may not have had anything to do with us. This is why we are called human beings, not human doings. It is the "being" part that is often left out of medicine and science. The intuitive aspects of the individual, the gut feeling that is not associated with what you ate, and the sense of knowing also needs acknowledgment – especially in scenarios of health *and* well-being. Being well is often thought of only from the perspective of the physical body. Well-being, however, is a sense, a feeling, and an experience of the intuitive energetic body.

In the next chapter, I will discuss this duality in depth and what we can learn from the yin/yang theory of TCM and how it relates to hypothyroid symptoms.

Diving Deeper

In TCM, we have five elements: wood, fire, earth, metal, and water. I also believe we have five bodies that bring perspective to our well-being. These bodies are not separate from each other. Instead, they are integrally intertwined and play off each other, much like yin and yang. If I were to draw them, they would look like Russian nesting dolls, but the reality is more like cake batter. One ingredient cannot be separated from another in the big picture, but an analysis can differentiate the components.

The first of these components is the *physical body*. We are all familiar with our physical body. Reach down and squeeze your thigh (without judgment); the point is not what that thigh feels like, but that you feel the physical presence of it. If you read the words and didn't do it, stop and squeeze please – there you go! Now, who is responsible for squeezing your thigh? If the answer in your head was anything other than "I am," we need to have a conversation on responsibility. You read the words on this page, written by the writer behind them, and the publisher who printed them, but no one else is there to make you do anything. Even though squeezing your thigh was suggested to you, you made a choice to squeeze or not to squeeze. The point is to start bringing awareness to your physical body, and the person behind the choice, who is not your body, but in the realm of mind.

Your *mind-body* is intimately connected to your brain, and your brain stores connections through something called synapses, or the loose connections between brain cells. We are programmed throughout our life with language, connections, and ideas and/or thoughts we or someone else had. Much of this programming is just that – a thought someone else had that we heard early in life and believed to be true. Some of these thoughts have been proven to be true, and someday they may be proven wrong, like the strongly held belief thousands of years ago that the world was flat. Today, that concept seems silly to us, as we know the earth is round, but it was the truth and reality most people held two thousand years ago. So, what I'm saying is that the programming of the mind-body can be changed, and in doing so, it also shifts the physical body.

Now, feel something toward anything or anyone you know. Feel love, anger, irritation, or admiration – the emotion itself doesn't matter, just feel it. This puts us in tune with our third body, the *emotional body*. Emotions have a different experience than thoughts, but thoughts bring about emotions. So, if you thought of your child and felt love, who is responsible for that feeling? "I am," is the answer again. Who is this "I am," if you are not your body, not your thought, and not your emotion? Who are you? This is the question that has been asked by philosophers, writers, and thinkers throughout history.

Have you ever had an experience where you think of a friend or loved one and then they call you? Often, this gets written off as coincidence. However, what if I were to tell you there is no coincidence? The thought is energetic in nature and not only did you hear or see a scenario in your mind, maybe feeling something throughout your body, but you also put out an energetic signal that your loved one received. Maybe you were the receiver of their thought, or maybe your thoughts were a simultaneous creation and they just picked up the phone first. This is your *energetic body*. Not only can we communicate with our physical body by typing, speaking, and using body language, but we can also communicate with thoughts and emotions on an energetic level. So, here is the question again, who is responsible for the signal to connect with your loved one? The voice in your head says, "I am," or maybe, "We are."

This "I am," when you clear away your body, thoughts, feelings, and all your humanness, is the being that is your higher Self. This is the spirit that you are when you are not weighed down by all of the responsibilities, programming, should, and roles humans create to keep busy and distracted. When you get back to just "being," it is often referred to as "bliss" and is experienced as an interconnectedness to all. For those who have had it, this experience is not sustainable long term. For a moment, we remember all our magnificence and then we forget. If you haven't had a moment of the magnificence and awe of what it is to be human "being," to be your Self, I sincerely hope that you do sometime soon.

For this book, we are going to refer to this fifth "body" as your higher Self or *spiritual body*. It has been referred to by many names and these glimpses of bliss are the reasoning behind most spiritual practices and spirituality, which is not to be confused with religion. Religions are their own entities that were originally formed to bring people together for spiritual practices. Today, the concepts can be collapsed, but churches and religion don't always incorporate spirituality, and there are many spiritual practices that have nothing to do with religion.

Downward causation is working with your higher Self through the energetic, emotional, and mind bodies to heal the physical body. Upward causation starts with the physical body and tries to work its

way upward into your mind, emotional, and energetic; this would
be like taking a drug of some sort to have a spiritual experience,
or for that matter, taking drugs and unnatural substance to "fix"
our problems. It doesn't work when it comes to actually healing
the whole being. Ideally, we work with the physical body to get
information about the other bodies and work toward whole healing.

Understanding the distinction of these five bodies is the
foundation of healing that makes what I describe in the rest of
the book a different approach than what you will find elsewhere.
Medicine only looks at the physical body, psychology primarily
addresses the mind-body and acknowledges that you have
emotions, but does not connect either with physical symptoms,
how it energetically impacts you, or spiritual existence. Spiritual
practices work on the spiritual body, but rarely do anything for
the physical or emotional. More traditional approaches like
shamanism, TCM and Ayurvedic (traditional medicine to India)
put together combinations of three or sometimes four of the
bodies, but do not speak of the five in relation to each other as I
do throughout the rest of this book.

So you have a place to flip back to for reference, here are the
five bodies:

- + Physical Body – Our biochemical processes, bones, tissues,
  and organs (the "particle")
- + Mind-Body – Our thoughts, learned beliefs, behaviors,
  and connections of concepts
- + Emotional Body – Our feelings and the waves and particles
  created in relation to them
- + Energetic Body – The reflection of our physical, but in
  energy form (the "wave")
- + Higher Self/Spiritual Body – The magnificent "God
  Spark"/soul that is defined by "I am"

CHAPTER 6

DUALITY

WHEN I WAS FIRST TAUGHT ABOUT YIN AND YANG, IT WAS spoken of in pairs of opposites and their dual nature, for example, hot and cold, dark and light, submissive and aggressive, dry and moist, day and night, active and still, and often referred to as the husband and wife. The point was not that each of these was exclusively yin or yang but that, by comparison, the part could only be truly understood by looking at the whole. Understanding that if we had never known light, dark would have no meaning and vice versa. However, in the light of day, there are always shadows, and in the darkness of night, there are always stars.

This logical comparison had certain truths; all things could be divided into two aspects, and that is further divided into two aspects that can then again be divided into two aspects, and so on. These two aspects seem to be in opposition to each other, hot versus cold, up versus down etc., but also depend on each other or mutually create and overtake the other. The absence of heat is cold; heat does not exist without cold, but cold is only known in the absence of heat. In a clinical sense, the patient with a high fever, if untreated, could go into shock and their body temperature drop. When we nourish our body with food, which is considered yin, our body uses it as energy for movement, which is yang. After an active day (yang), the body needs rest (yin). The yin is consumed by yang and eventually returns to a state of yin.

Throughout the written texts, there are numerous variations about what is considered yang and what is considered yin based on one of the original stories where the emperor held a conference in which he stood in the North, facing the crowd of people. He pointed to the East and said, "The sun rises in the East; this is yang. The sun sets in the West; this is yin." As any good leader would do, the emperor lifted his left arm for the East and right for the West. This is often interpreted to mean that left is yang and right is yin. However, this intuitively makes no sense when you add in the fact that yang is considered the active – the giving, the doing, and the outward and upward aspects of movement that the majority of the population does with our right hand.

In the story, I think they made a point of saying that the emperor stood in the North, at the head of the body of people, for a reason. The only logical and intuitive explanation is that the emperor is the representation of the brain in relation to the body or body of people. In this sense, the left-brain characteristics of logic, directness, and linear thinking control the right side of the body, whereas the right side of the brain is creative, receptive to new ideas, and often less organized, controls the left side of the body. This belief is reflected in chart below:

Yang	Yin
Masculine	Feminine
Logical	Creative
Linear	Curvy or round about
Active	Passive
Left Brain	Right Brain
Right side of Body	Left side of Body
Thinking	Feeling
Doing	Being
Logical	Intuitive
Seen	Unseen
Physiological	Spiritual
Math and science	Artistic expression
Analysis and breaking things down	Imagination and making things up
"The way things are"	"What is possible"
Day	Night
Fast	Slow
Upper	Lower
Exertion	Nourishment
Exterior	Interior
Giving	Receiving
Studying	Experiencing
Bowels	Organs
Leaner	Fatter
Lighter	Heavier
Rigid	Flexible
Stronger (physically)	Weaker
Testosterone (progesterone)	Estrogen
Awake	Asleep
Work	Rest
Money	Love
Respect	Appreciation, gratitude
Surgery, bloodwork, medications	Meditation, prayer, energy healing
Brain	Mind-Body
Emotions (brain chemicals)	Feelings (the sensations); empathy
Upward causation	Downward causation

Gender roles go out the window when you consider that we all have all of this within us. Some relate with one more than the other, but as the symbol suggests, even the most logical thinker can come up with something out of the box and the most creative intuitive can balance their checkbook with some focus and effort. Yin gives rise to yang every day in every way, just as the sun rises and sets.

Over the years, what I noticed with my patients was that their physical bodies would give us insight, or a road map, to where those "unseen" answers were. If all of their pain was on their right (yang), they generally struggled with physical or "work" related issues (work could mean exercise, actual work in the workplace, or the way our body works to break things down). On the other hand, if most of the pain they experienced was on the left (yin), it would suggest more emotional aspects or a block in creativity or self-expression.

Think of this like a dialogue in its own language. Your body tells you specifically what is going on, but you don't have the language to understand it yet. It could be as simple as a food craving, like chocolate – specifically dark chocolate. This craving is not just a preference, but that gentle nudge of, "I could use a piece of dark chocolate right now." Most people either eat the chocolate or don't and move on without a second thought. However, if you know that most cravings for dark chocolate are associated with the body needing more magnesium, you might eat more foods with magnesium or take a supplement.

Hypothyroid symptoms, cold, tired, puffy, sluggish, and foggy-brained are all considered yin. Hyperthyroid symptoms, hot, anxious, weight loss, rapid heartbeat, and difficulty sleeping, are all considered yang. If we start to consider that all of these yin symptoms are either an excess of yin or a lack of yang, we will want to look at internal aspects of function; are we overnourished or underactive? Are we not being able to create the thyroid hormone because a lack of nourishment (yin) or a breakdown in the process of work (yang)? Are we overrun with estrogen (from birth control or phytoestrogens) or deficient of testosterone/progesterone? Are we holding onto things emotionally or receiving everyone else's stuff (empathy)? Are we emptying the bowels properly and nourishing the organs? Sometimes, the answer to these questions is both. An example of this is the thirty-year-old patient who has been on birth control for over a decade and does not break down estrogen very well. This excess yin initially causes a relative lack of progesterone (yang) preventing pregnancy but, over time, creates a deficiency of progesterone and testosterone and extremely high estrogen (yin).

Using intuition, getting the patient's own intuitive feedback and awareness of symptoms is the best diagnostic tool for truly integrative medicine. The pursuit of health and well-being is a lifelong journey that is made easier when you have a common language to work with. Traditional Chinese medicine has given us many tools to work with, but I am expanding that base by adding and bringing science to the table as well.

The next five chapters dive into the five elements of TCM: wood, fire, earth, metal, and water. Each element has aspects of each of the five bodies – physical, energetic, emotional, mind and spiritual.

Each will have a section of the physical and energetic body, mind-body, emotional body and spiritual practice to bring balance to the others. The physical and energetic bodies are written together as they are the yin/yang of Qi itself. It is like heads and tails of a coin. You can't really discuss one that is not relevant to the other, nor can you see the opposite when looking at one side unless you are looking at that one side in front of a mirror where you can see the other reflected back to you. I invite you to read it all and reread the sections that aren't as easy for you, put them into practice and sit with them as long as you need to. This is a great opportunity to get in touch with community reading this as well. It is much easier for others to show you your reflection than trying to see your blind spots in a mirror by yourself. There will be left-brained logical thinkers who want to skip straight to the doing and right-brained creatives who want to skip the science all together. It is likely that the areas you don't want to spend time with will provide you with your best answers.

CHAPTER 7

HEALTHY DETOX –
THE WOOD ELEMENT

THE ELEMENT OF WOOD CAPTURES MANY ASPECTS OF TREES. Trees grow and are flexible and strong; their canopy offers safety, and from it, you can see far. Trees clean up the environment around them, while protecting what is under their shelter from damage and so much more. Their smell is clean and fresh and cut wood is a little sour. Many trees go through cycles of growth and rest, blooming and shedding. Trees are nourished by water, sunlight, and nutrients from the earth (minerals). If nutrients or water is missing, trees become weak or brittle and can wither and break.

Physical and Energetic Body

In our bodies, we look for similar characteristics to trees. Our tendons and ligaments are also flexible and strong; our eyes allow us to see far, and our liver cleans up and protects us from environmental toxins while producing bile to break down and make use of the foods we've eaten. The taste of sour is associated with the wood element and many of the herbs that treat it are considered sour. Our liver also produces bile, a sour substance that breaks down fat from our diet.

Children tend to have active liver energy as they grow. Children are more flexible, not just in their tendons and ligaments, but also in their bones, muscles, and minds. Additionally, their love of sour candy is one expression of the relationship to growth, sour taste, and the wood element. Our bodies require nutrients for our liver to do its job of detoxification and protect us from the environment. Without these nutrients, our tendons become dry, and our fingernails, which are considered excess tendon in TCM, begin to flake, peel, break, and deform. Women's bodies also have a blooming and shedding effect with our monthly cycles, making the wood element one of the elements used in treatment of fertility and women's health. Without sunlight, we do not make vitamin D3. Vitamin D is actually a hormone that has numerous functions in the body and has shown to benefit energy and sleep quality.

The partner to the liver is the gallbladder, and its job is to store bile for when the body is in a rest and digest state. In TCM, we say the liver maintains the free flow of Qi, stores the blood, controls tendons, manifests nails, and opens into the eyes. As we discussed earlier, Qi refers to the wave/particle form of the ion and biochemical processes, and the liver itself is responsible for over five hundred different biochemical processes done thousands of times a day. These processes are considered yang, as they are active, heat-creating functions. The liver energy is said to be most easily affected by stagnation and stress. When we think of stress, most of us think of emotional stress. But weather and temperature changes, pollens in the air, chemicals in our environment, not enough sleep, too much food, happy events, sad events, reaction to news, and not enough time to process our experiences are all forms of stress that impact us on an energetic, emotional, and even physical level. The mind is generally not even aware of the majority of these stressors. Then we add the ones we are aware of like the job, situations, and people that "stress us out."

There is no easy way to say this, but we live in a toxic world. Most people don't realize how often they encounter chemicals, many of which are toxic to our bodies. A recent study looked at infants' cord blood born that day and found an average of two hundred chemicals in the blood that would not have been there fifty to one hundred years ago. This comes from the fact that most women are exposed to more than two hundred chemicals before breakfast, as they use shampoo, conditioner, lotions, gels, face creams, deodorant, hair spray, perfumes, and cosmetics that are loaded with unnecessary chemical compounds that were not used fifty to one hundred years ago. The average woman is completely unaware of the impact this can have on her health or that of an unborn child. No one anywhere teaches us to read the ingredient list of these sorts of products, much less what to make of it, so we assume they are safe. Most of us don't put a second thought to putting these products on the outside of our body. After all, if it smells good and makes our hands softer, isn't it doing its job? Our skin absorbs the products we use, including all those chemicals, many of which can be toxic in excess, and our liver has the task of ridding our body of them.

If the chemicals stopped there, we might not be overloaded, but it doesn't, because I haven't even mentioned what we eat or breathe. Processed foods are also loaded with chemicals, colors, and preservatives that sometimes are even labeled "natural." What companies don't tell you is that "natural" doesn't mean that your body can process it or that it is good for you. Let's face it, arsenic is an all-natural compound that can be found naturally in peach pits and other stone fruits, and we all know that it can kill you if too much is ingested. So, why would we purposefully eat something like arsenic – or even a peach pit, for that matter? You wouldn't, yet you do every day in foods like rice, fruits, vegetables, and fish; even by drinking water. Arsenic has been used across industries, including in ore mines, pesticides, to make copper products, to preserve wood, for semiconductor devices, and for lead and glass alloys. The point here isn't to pick on arsenic; rather, the point is that even known poisons that we wouldn't choose to be exposed to are all over our environment and we don't even know it. Our bodies can manage very tiny amounts as they come to us naturally, but when larger amounts sneak into our bodies because of pollution and industrial overuse, we more easily become affected by all chemicals. Becoming more aware of the biggest offenders that we can control to a certain extent, we are able to take off some of the load and reduce the stress on our body. Phthalates (found in plastics are hormone disruptors), glyphosate (herbicide most heavily used in grains, but on many fruits and vegies as well), and other common chemicals in our environment can be avoided or at least minimized by dietary and lifestyle choices. Learning what they are and how to avoid them, helps us become more proactive in our own health care. Buying organic where available, growing your own vegetables or fruits, and buying from local farmers who can tell you what chemicals were used or not are ways to clean up pesticide and herbacide exposure in your diet. Limiting the use of Styrofoam and plastic containers and water bottles reduces exposure to phthalates. Glass and stainless-steel cups are readily available in most stores. This also requires us to slow down and eat with consciousness. Drive-throughs are not going to offer minimal exposure to these toxins in most cases. There have been a few changes in some restaurants of using paper straws instead of plastic ones and more environmentally friendly paper cups, but that is not the majority. Awareness and personal choice at the individual level will shape the future of what is available for our children and future generations.

Our bodies are wise and designed to protect us against micro-exposures to these types of chemicals. However, between pollution in our air, and chemicals in everything we do, touch, and eat, we are in a constant onslaught that many bodies struggle to keep up with. This is when we start to develop the beyond adaptation fatigue stage that I mentioned in Chapter 4, and this toxic overload is at the source of hypothyroid, type-II diabetes, MS flare ups, chronic inflammation and pain, and the precursors for cancer and many of our other current chronic health problems.

Think of it like this – if our body was a factory producing cars, we know that each step in the factory requires a certain quantity of a particular part, like four wheels and four tires, a front and back bumper, one engine, one steering wheel, seven parts of the frame, whatever exact number of bolts and nuts, and so on. If you want to make sixteen cars that day, you need sixteen times what was listed in the "ingredients," and each of those stations needs to be functioning properly. Imagine the first ten cars came out perfectly, but the ones after that weren't functioning properly. Do you say the manufacturing is bad and build another factory, or do you go look for what went wrong? Were there not enough steering wheels, nuts, bolts, or tires, or was there actually a problem with the station at which those were put on?

Most often, we blame the station when it comes to our health, like the thyroid or our other hormone-producing parts, for not doing their job. Instead of putting in more parts that are necessary for function at the station with which they are needed, we add an extra station at the end that replaces the whole car with one from another factory. It makes no sense. Most likely, your factory – your body – is fine; it is stressed from environmental load and a lack of quality nutrients.

The Science and Medicine of the Wood Element

In medicine, phase I and phase II liver detox, which help us rid the body of toxins, are biochemical processes your body does without your knowledge. You don't have to think, "Okay, liver, it's time to break down those chemicals and take out the trash." It does however, require a variety of B vitamins; iron; antioxidants, like vitamins C and E; and magnesium indoles (chemical compounds-natural) from cruciferous vegetables like broccoli. Phase II requires sulfur-containing foods like onions, leeks, shallots, raw garlic, eggs, and cruciferous vegetables (broccoli, brussels sprouts, cabbage, cauliflower). Phase I liver detox breaks down the toxins into intermediate substances that are neutralized in phase II and excreted in either feces or urine. All of these steps are dependent on each other, and if phase I is rapid and phase II slow, there can be a buildup of intermediary molecules, some of which are harmless and some of which can be inflammatory or carcinogenic. Curcumin, which is found in the spice turmeric, slows down phase I and speeds up phase II, helping people with inflammation from these intermediaries process more evenly. Ideally, we would get these vitamins, minerals and compounds like curcumin from our diet, but it may be necessary in the short term to supplement higher dosages of some of these nutrients to help along the detoxing of an overloaded system. Once, we get back to a less toxic state it may still be necessary to supplement at lower dosages to maintain homeostasis or a state of balance. It is unfortunate that our farming processes over the years have depleted soil where commercial produce is grown and even beautiful produce on the shelf at the grocery store doesn't supply us with the nutrients they once did.

So, how do you know if your phase I or II is faster or slower or in need of support? This is where genetics comes in. We all have single nucleotide pairs (SNPs), often called snips, that vary throughout our genetic material. Some of us work faster, slower, or don't conjugate certain vitamins or other nutrients as well as others. While this is something that can be looked into for the curious using DNA testing and someone to help interpret the findings, it isn't necessary to know and understand for you to feel much better. You can feel improved health with a shift in diet and lifestyle and when necessary, to speed up or support that process, quality activated supplements that are targeted and specific to you. It is estimated that up to 95 percent of our health problems are environmental, not genetic. Even when your parents, grandparents, or siblings all have the same issue, it is likely that you do share a SNP or many that cause similar symptoms to a toxic environment that you all live in similarly. When the body is under stress or the type of chemical load I referred to, disease-producing SNPs are turned on like a light switch. They can be turned off when the body is no longer under stress and allowed to function at its own pace with proper nutrients. This is why diet and lifestyle are so important. Doing a fad diet for three months may make you feel better and lose weight, but after you quit, you end up going right back to where you started or worse. Too many of these diets are meant to produce quick results and are not sustainable. Sustainable changes come over time and are processes, they are choices you can live with for the rest of your life.

Ideally, we support both phases of liver detox by cleaning up our personal environment the best we can by what we eat and what we expose ourselves to. When you run out of the blue perfume-laden laundry detergent, try one that is free and clear of some of the chemicals and dyes and replace your dryer sheets with wool dryer balls and essential oils; these actions alone cut out numerous hormone-disrupting chemicals. Eat more organic fruits and vegies, especially ones that are on the EWG.org "Dirty Dozen" list. I will put an action list at the end of the chapter providing you with lists of changes that can easily be done at home to help yourselves.

Emotional Body

Other yin aspects of the elements are all about the waves of emotion, the unseen processes of the emotional body. I think of e-motions like energy ("e" is also the connotation for the electron) in motion, where the motion is yang to the overall yin aspect of emotions. Some of my scientist friends like to mark emotions up to only physiological processes that are biochemical in nature and made just like other particles in our body in reaction to connections in the brain. I try to be nice, because I understand what my friends are saying, but I also feel things so deeply and strongly and am acutely aware of textures, the expansion, and the contraction of my energetic body in response to emotions that it is hard for me to believe that our emotions are only physiological processes. More so, I believe that emotions are part of the way our spirit communicates with our physical body and that we are all capable of not only sensing our own emotions but are also able to sense others' emotions. Much like anything in life, some of us are more attuned to others' emotions and feel them more strongly. Those of us who are more sensitive to others' emotions probably heard as a child that they were just "too sensitive," or were told to stop crying it's not a big deal, or even worse "if you don't stop crying, I'll give you something to cry about." Therefore, we learned to stuff our emotions, swallow our anger, or just ignore that gut feeling, grief, and sadness. I'm here to tell you that as an adult, when you see those sensitivities as a guidance system and embrace them as one of your greatest gifts, not only will you grow in confidence, strength, and power, but you will also start to notice that your symptoms often correspond to your experiences.

As a young acupuncturist, I started to notice that when speaking of the emotional aspects of TCM with my patients, their bodies started to shift toward healing. Even if they didn't open up and express what was bothering them, knowing that what they were experiencing had reason gave them a little freedom. That emotion coming to the surface before or during an acupuncture session often gave them a much greater experience of healing.

The wood element in TCM is most easily affected by stress. In the yang aspects, we saw that environmental stressors weigh heavily on the actual liver and its processes, where the emotional stressors affect the yin aspects of the emotional and energetic bodies. I can't tell you how many times over the years I have reached to feel my patient's pulse and their arm is extended straight out in the air. I tell my patients to relax, and they say, "I am," yet their arm is still tensely extended in midair. I gently shake their wrist and say "relax" again.

Most patients say, "Oh," and let go of the tension in their arm so that it relaxes next to them on the table. This is a constant reminder of how much we have adapted to our stress. That tension is not normal; we don't have to hold ourselves out for others all the time. Sometimes, we think it is polite to be so on guard and vigilant, but it works against you in the long run.

The wood element, specifically the liver channel in TCM is primarily associated with the emotion of anger. I also associate liver with varying degrees of anger, such as irritability, frustration, rage, suppression of emotions, and depression. The gallbladder is associated with decision-making and "the nerve of you" reaction when someone proverbially steps on your toes or even an amount of courage in taking a bold action. The aspects of the gallbladder apply whether you have had yours surgically removed or not; the physical removal of the GB is of minimal consequence to the meridian or emotion itself, but the emotions may have been a contributor for the need to have it removed.

In working with low-grade depression associated with hypothyroid symptoms, I invite you to ask yourself how often you suppress your emotions, particularly anger, and noting when it started. Growing up in a household with a postwar veteran who often had angry outbursts, I know that I decided at an early age that I didn't like anger; anger scared me, and I didn't like the way it felt, even when it was directed at someone else. I didn't like being around it or people who were angry often; I didn't like feeling like I wanted to hit or hurt someone. However, I did feel that way at times and I shut it down, pushed it down, and covered it with a smile. I swallowed my own angry reactions because that's what "good girls" were expected to do, and as I got older it was one of the ways I felt like kept me "safe."

"Don't let them see they've gotten to you; don't fight back. Just hold your chin up and keep going," was my mother's advice when dealing with mean girls at school. You can start to see by the language that we use when speaking of anger that is something that rises up, we call this flaring of liver fire; it is also often seen in the red face, nose or eyes of alcoholics. You can also start to understand that swallowing anger down is the opposite of the emotion itself. Anger is expansive, it rises upward and increases the overall vibration of the body. So often, when someone comes in with a sore throat, the first question I ask is if they swallowed their anger lately. You would be amazed how many people think I'm psychic, when it is their body doing the talking. When we learn to feel the expansion and sit in the emotion and heightened vibration without expelling the energy on some object or verbally throwing it at others in the form of blame, something else becomes available in the form of a higher perspective and "right" action. This is not to be confused with moral right and wrong, but a higher guidance that moves forward a situation for what is in the best interest and highest good of all involved.

To me, frustration feels more like someone bumping up against the edge of their box. I think we all have a box or a glass ceiling that, as we grow and change spiritually, we bump up against. It often takes bumping up against the box and the frustration of it to get angry, expand passed our box, and see a higher perspective. Unfortunately, for many people, it is too easy to expel our anger on others, point fingers, play the blame game, and continue to stay in this small box we created for ourselves. Many people survive here for years, and that survival and blame instead of growth and expansion leads to more depression, suppression, and anger until it becomes bitterness, which is actually an emotion associated with the element of fire, which is up next.

The Mind-Body

The mind-body in the wood element is about ego. This is not necessarily the arrogance, "chip on the shoulder" ego, but the identity that you created through life experiences, the roles you play, and the meanings that you made from those experiences and roles. What are some of the roles you play? Are you a mom, sister, daughter, healer, provider, friend, or confidant? The list could go on.

We often say, "I am his/her mom." and while it is true that you had a child or adopted one, you are you, a powerful individual being who has taken on the responsibility of guiding another powerful individual. Historically, in our culture, women and children were treated like possessions to own and force into submission or roles. I, for one, am grateful that this is no longer the case. As someone who's been on this planet for numerous decades, I recognize that while this is better, we still see the struggle to control others or not be controlled by others in everything from TV and politics to the way corporations and households are run. Most commercials and marketing are designed to control your thoughts on something in order to get you to buy a product. This plays on your ego and identity to make you want to be more like the "good" mom, or whatever is portrayed in the commercial. Being able to see through the hype and discern some level of truth is an action of vision associated with the wood element. Sometimes just having a new awareness of this is enough to start the conversation with yourself of what is ego and what isn't. Oftentimes, though, getting to a healthy place with your ego takes introspection and looking at where in the past those identities may have come from.

As children, life experiences happen; you played with your best friend and wanted to go to the swings, but she wanted to go somewhere else and did so with another friend. You might have thought this meant your friend didn't like you anymore or liked someone else more. However, the truth was that you wanted one thing, and she wanted another – it had nothing to do with being less liked than the other kids. It is human nature to make meaning out of our world. It is the things we believe to be true about our Self that we have to look at; often, it's just what we came to believe in our mind and created as part of our ego. When you find yourself in reaction to a situation, it is a beneficial tool to take a step back, look at what actually happened, and ask, "What, if anything, did I make it mean about me or the other person?"

Did an experience trigger something you decided about yourself many years ago? Specifically, when it comes to anger as the reaction, what was your expectation that was unmet? Was it a communicated expectation? The more practice you have with understanding your own mind, the quicker you will be able to notice and let go of those reactions.

To give you an example of understanding this, when I was born, my father's business had burned to the ground with no insurance compensation. My mother had just left her job so she could stay home with me and my brother, and she injured her back. It caused her a great deal of pain to lift me from the crib, so when my dad left for work early, he would take me out and lay me on a pallet on the floor. As infants, we are extra sensitive to energies and aware of much more than we are given credit for. I can imagine that when

I cried for my mother, it caused her a great deal of pain to get on the floor to feed, change, or interact with me.

When I came to understand this dynamic, it brought light to why I had always felt like "I hurt the people I cared for" or that I couldn't ask for help because it would hurt others to do that for me. This was a pattern that seemed to show up for me in relationships, friendships, or any other time I expected someone else to help me, such as during group projects in college.

Now, being an acupuncturist, how do you think this sort of belief about myself worked? It didn't. I struggled to get patients in the beginning; when I did get them, I was nervous I would hurt them, so I wouldn't use the full extent of my knowledge. And I had no support because I wouldn't ask for it. I came to realize that this was one of the many things that held me back in practice, business, and life, so I was able to make a "quantum shift" in my way of being. This type of mind-set work helps us to create freedom where we have been stuck.

Mind-set impacts Qi, much like the observer in the experiment mentioned in Chapter 5. Our stuck emotions, or in this chapter, the anger pushed down or the tears swallowed are how we take a wave of emotion and stop it where it is putting it into particle form. We often do this without conscious observation of what it feels like in our body. Most that do this, have had the experience of tightness in their throat. That tightness is where the energy is stopped or stuck. It is also where your thyroid is. Someone with a goiter or swollen thyroid may have a similar experience of thickness or tightness in their throat. I'm not saying that all goiters are caused by suppression of anger, I am saying that this pattern over time contributes to the stress of the body and focuses it right where the person with hypothyroid feels "pain." In TCM there is an old phrase "When there is free flow of Qi there is no pain; pain exists when there is no free flow."

Putting It All Together

You may have heard the saying "As above, so below" from the religious perspective at one time or another, but what does it mean? In this sense, I think of it like a projection. All of the stuff you have from mind-body and emotional-body is like clothing to your energetic body. You wrap yourself in the mom robe, the sisterhood pants, the teacher dress, the disliked kid costume, the weird scientist hat, the rock-star wanna-be T-shirt, the failed project cloak of shame, a suit of armor, and the list just keeps going for every experience and identity you once had. You have on so many outfits that you are weighed down; no wonder you are tired.

With all of the information bombarding you from a culture that tries to tell you who and how you should be, not to mention the fabulous Facebook lives all your friends have, how do you ever unwind your own insane outfit to possibly make sense of any of it? You do so one step at a time, one day at a time, and you can be assured that all those other people out there have on crazy outfits too.

Your body and mind have basically put on the brakes and forced you to slow down with symptoms of fatigue and lethargy. You can only process so much stuff at once and the pace at which we have been living life is too much for most. Much like your liver can only process so many chemicals and toxins, your energetic body can only process and filter so much input as well. Interestingly enough, your physical body is not just a reflection of your energetic body, but also a reflection of our planet, and in the wood element, this reflects our forests and plant growth. How can we possibly maintain the rate of growth and expansion with the current level of toxicity and disrespect for our bodies and forests?

The Higher Self

In the element of wood, access to this higher consciousness of ourselves often comes from righteous anger. That may be off-putting to read, and it is the reason that most people do not access higher consciousness in this way. Remember earlier when I said that frustration was bumping up against the box that we created, meaning our ego? We can either work through the mind-body to deconstruct meanings in our ego and/or through the emotional body. In the emotional body, anger helps us expand past that ego box, but many people expel their anger and blame others. This is *not* the action of higher Self. The action of higher Self in this element is to use our anger as an indicator for personal growth, to rise above the current circumstances and see a better way. To see injustice, let anger be a building block to serenity and purpose. This makes me think of movies like *The Hunger Games* and *X-Men*. In *The Hunger Games*, the lead character is fueled by righteous anger, giving her focus and purpose that she can only achieve by dealing with her own emotions and identity to the point of being willing to sacrifice her life to make a difference for her people. In one of the *X-Men* movies, a young Xavier tells his best friend that his power lies in finding the serenity in the midst of all his anger, to focus it, and then to let go.

Most of the people in our society are so busy with all of the "doing" and keeping up that they will never experience the kind of purpose and passion that fuels this type of power. Yet, you can reclaim your own energy and power by seeing what your bodies (physical, emotional, mind) react to, finding your own serenity in it, and then, with purpose, taking action. The gift of the wood element to the higher Self is that of extraordinary vision, and I don't mean twenty-twenty vision; I mean the kind of vision that sees a problem, asks what is possible, and is able to see something new for themselves and others. And the wisdom to know what is actionable and what is not.

To get there, we start by cleaning up our diet so our physical body can be clear and energetic, clearing our mind of the shoulds, expectations, and ideas of who we are, dealing with our own emotions and expectations of those around us, and lessening the load of the energetic body by starting to see where we carry a load that no longer serves us and likely wasn't even ours to carry in the first place. Last but not least, start visualizing what you want things to be like.

Actions to Take

For the Physical Body in Your Environment

1. Start switching out cleaning and laundry products with cleaner versions that have less chemicals, dyes, and artificial scents. Most everyday cleaners can be made at home with vinegar, water, baking soda, and essential oils for a fraction of the cost of store-bought products. Pinterest has a wealth of recipes and ideas. Detergents can be a little tricky to make at home, but cleaner versions are easily available. On our website there are pages you can download to start making these changes over the next 6 months.

2. Don't get overwhelmed. This is a process, not something to overhaul all at once! As your personal care products come to an end, look for cleaner, more environmentally friendly versions. You may have to try several products over time to find out what works best for you. We have some examples of cleaner lines on our website.

3. Go to EWG.org and print off or take a picture of the "Dirty Dozen, Clean 15" lists. Only eat the items on the

"Dirty Dozen" list if they are organic, if they are not, just skip them and eat something else. The "Clean 15" list can be bought and eaten safely, if the items are non-GMO (genetically modified).

4. Cut out wheat, not because wheat is bad for everyone, or because gluten is terrible, but because it is one of the highest contaminated foods with glyphosate. It is standard protocol that before wheat is cut to be brought in from the field, it is sprayed heavily with Roundup to kill and dry up any weeds that don't belong there. Glyphosate has been linked to numerous kinds of cancers and other health problems. Some of the products with highest concentrations of glyphosate are Cheerios and Goldfish; if you want these types of foods for your children, buy the organic ones.

5. Start switching out nonstick cookware with glass, stainless steel, or cast iron. The nonstick coating is heavy in phthalates and other carcinogenic materials when aged, damaged, or flaking

For the Energetic Body in Your Environment

1. Start noticing the feel of rooms when you walk in. Does the clutter make you contract? As you look around do you feel stopped by something out of place or odd? Does it feel relaxing and serene? Taking notice of your space starts to help you make shifts in your physical environment that impact your energetic, spiritual and mind bodies that in turn help the physical body feel less stressed and on guard.

2. Notice when you go to the grocery store or other shopping if you feel rushed, overwhelmed, dirty, or at ease. If what you feel isn't pleasant to you, consider shopping elsewhere.

3. Notice in the presence of friends and family how you feel. And how you feel once they are gone. This will give you clues to where some of your stuck energy and stories come from.

For the Emotional Body

Give yourself a quiet space to relax and consider these questions, without distractions or interruptions:

1. How often do I feel blah, in a funk, or depressed?
2. Who am I around when I feel this way? (or, who was I just around or on the phone with?)
3. What situation did I just leave? (e.g., grocery store, mall, school event, work)
4. When I feel angry (consider questions 2 and 3 here too), did I have an unmet expectation? Was that expectation communicated clearly? What if anything is the next best step? If you swallowed your anger, take notice of how it felt in your physical body. If you blamed another, how does it feel to notice the impact your blame had on them? If you don't know what that impact was on them, ask them when you have both cooled off.
5. When you feel frustrated, what do you do about it? (Consider 2 and 3) Do you throw up your hands and say this is the way it always goes? Do you go take a nap? Do you consider what else is possible?

These may seem irrelevant in the short term, but the more aware you become of your emotions and how you work with them, the more aware you will become of how they affect your overall symptoms and where you lose energy or give it over to others.

For the Mind-Body

1. Make a list of the rolls you play in life as I am statements: I am a daughter, I am a teacher, I am a…

2. Now envision an outfit for each and make note of it.

3. Start noticing when you have on what outfit and how it makes you feel. Some are more empowering than others. Take one situation and outfit at a time, as they occur to you. This is a process. Uncovering who you are without all the ego identity is an ongoing endeavor.

4. If that outfit no longer serves you, you wear it in the wrong situations too often, or you are just ready to update it, imagine burning it, throwing it away or taking it off and retiring it in whatever way works for you.

5. Once you've let go of an outfit create an "I am" statement that empowers you: I am love (loved or loving), I am wise, I am strong, courageous, whatever you want to feel that is not a role you play.

6. Moving forward if you find yourself slipping back into a roll, remind yourself of your statement of affirmation. Or just use "I am loved, I am worthy and I am whole and complete just as I am."

This exercise helps us to unload some of the weight we put on over time in our life (physically, energetically, and emotionally). When we are weighed down by our past, our body continues to react to our present as if those situations are still threatening, even if they weren't really threats to begin with.

An example: I am the little sister. My outfit is a hand-me-down sweatshirt from my older brother with my hair in messy pigtails. I feel competitive and like I can outdo and win if I just weren't so much smaller and winning means I am more loved. So, I might just be more cunning, even mean, to get one over on him and win. I'm hyper aware of pointing out flaws and when he breaks the rules. I recognize that I was probably three or four when I put this one on. I envision taking off the sweatshirt, stepping into my adult self, and letting go of the past. I create the statements I am love, I am kind, I am wise, I am enough. In this scenario, being love, kind, wise, and enough replaces the need to outdo big brother and creates space for something else to be present.

CHAPTER 8

THE MIND, SLEEP, AND GETTING CONNECTED – THE FIRE ELEMENT

THE ELEMENT OF FIRE IS AS MYSTERIOUS AS FIRE ITSELF. WE all know the beautiful, mesmerizing flicker of flames, but this yellow-orange apparition is barely a hint to the invisible fire that rages below, and the reach of heat created by it. Fire is swift and unpredictable. It is the element that binds things together or softens them to become moldable. Fire can rage or smolder. It is often associated with passion and warmth, but when out of control it is associated with devastating destruction. Fire cleanses by burning away anything in its path and returning it to ash and earth.

Physical and Energetic Body

In traditional Chinese medicine, the element of fire is also filled with mystery. It is associated with the heart, pericardium, small intestine, and something called the San Jiao (translated as "triple burner"). In the physical body, we know that the heart is the muscle that pumps blood through the vascular system (veins, capillaries, arteries), and the pericardium is the lining around the heart that protects it. This is also recognized in TCM, but they take it further by saying, "The heart houses the mind," "opens to the tongue and face," and that "sweat is the fluid of the heart." In TCM, the heart is the monarch of all organs, and the taste associated with it is bitter. The mind, in this scenario, refers to both the conscious and subconscious mind existence, and it is closely associated with the ability to sleep. When we cannot rest to recover, none of our organs function optimally. The busy brain can't fall asleep, so some may experience insomnia as a dysfunction of the fire element, particularly heart and pericardium. Hypothyroid patients vary on how their sleep quality is, even if they are tired all the time, doesn't mean they are getting enough sleep, or quality sleep, which further compounds the fatigue they feel.

The small intestine is responsible for separating the clear from the turbid (cloudy, unclear, dirty); it is responsible for discernment, clarity, and the sorting and moving away of turbidity. We see the small intestine as the long tube that helps us continue to break down foods and separate out the useful from the waste. In the functional medicine community, the environment of the small intestine has gotten a lot of attention with the continued understanding of the microbiome and its dysfunction in cases of SIBO (small intestine bacterial overgrowth). In TCM, the small intestine also follows the pathways in the arm and shoulder blade that can be quite painful in cases of rotator cuff injury and frozen shoulder. Foggy brain and an inability to make decisions may also be due to the body needing time to sort out the turbidity of food and/or life experiences.

The San Jiao (triple burner) is the most mysterious aspect of this fabulous four, in the fact that no one has any real evidence for what it refers to physiologically. The texts speak of a separation above the diaphragm (upper jiao), between the diaphragm and umbilicus (middle jiao), and below the umbilicus (lower jiao). Other than interstitial fluid, that ideally creates a slippery surface for our organs to avoid sticking together, there seems to be no physical evidence for such a thing. It seems to be used more for harmony between the systems and to clear up or "dredge the internal pathways" to keep things flowing and moving smoothly.

In medicine and TCM, dysfunctions of the heart often occur because of fire flaring, or inflammation, in conjunction with blockages in the vessels, often caused by cholesterol getting stuck to the inflamed walls of the vessels. More and more research over the last twenty years has shown that heart disease is a function of inflammation, not necessarily cholesterol numbers. Containing or controlling inflammation (fire) is the key to physical heart health, and there are specific tests that look at inflammation and cholesterol balance as indicators for heart health.

The Science and Medicine of Sleep

Sleep is one of the most important things we can do for our bodies. Oftentimes, lack of quality sleep is at the source of fatigue, brain fog, mild depression, and even weight gain. While sleeping, our conscious and subconscious minds integrate; our tissues repair; memory, learning, and mood are regulated; and mental restoration is promoted. In modern times, as we are bombarded with information, it is often hard to shut off to get to sleep. Not to mention, we face unusually high amounts of blue light that we get from all of our little screens, which trick our brains into thinking that it is still light out even when the sun set hours ago. One of the best things we can do for ourselves is to shut off the blue lights and little screens at least thirty minutes before bedtime. There are increasing numbers of studies about the effects of computer screen time and brain development in children, as well as the effects of sleep patterns in adults. If you have a busy brain that just won't shut off, even though you feel exhausted, or your brain reminds you of the same things over and over, get a journal to put by your bed. Once you turn of the screens, spend that thirty minutes dumping all of those thoughts onto paper so they are out of your head. If you wake up in the middle of the night and need to do it again, write more, but try to find a red light to use, as it promotes sleep in the brain much like a sunset signals the end of the day.

We often find the heart and the brain at war with each other. Do you follow your heart or listen to your head? The heart actually has sixty times the electromagnetic charge of the brain. In fact, it is measurably the strongest electrical impulse in the entire body. We generate our electromagnetism from the heart. When we speak of attraction, electromagnetically, that comes from the heart. Too often, as we all know, our brain gets in the way.

Mind-Body

Meditation is one of the best ways to get back to our own heart center in connection with our spirit. A sensitive person who lives with others is often bombarded with everyone else's emotions, thoughts, and unseen energies. Taking time by yourself to sit, center, and breathe is one of the quickest ways to get back to a happy heart instead of a busy brain, even if this time means taking an extra three to five minutes in the shower as the water washes over you. Close your eyes, let the water wash away and cleanse all that is not yours from you. Recenter into your heart space and choose joy for the day, knowing that all of the cacophony of the world is not yours and you don't have to fix it, change it, or make it all better. All you have to do is be – be you; it is more than enough. What I notice when I do this often is an overall better sense of well-being, being more grounded and more available to respond to situations around me at the time and the wisdom to know when it's not my place to step in and do something about it. This may seem minor or unrelated to thyroid, but when your energy is low, determining what actions are the best use of the energy you have reserves all the energy we use on stuff that doesn't really matter.

The fire element is all about relationships. If those relationships are toxic, it reflects in your liver and body. Many people choose to drown that sadness with alcohol or other further damaging drugs that take us further away from our heart center. As wood is fire's fuel, these elements are impossible to view completely separate of each other. Rage is the fire fueled by wood, or some version of passion fueled by anger. Unlike our medical system, in which you would have different doctors for your heart and every other organ system, traditional Chinese medicine teaches that all organs are interconnected and depend on each other's processes. This recognition alone brings order to a chaotic medical system that sends you to multiple specialists for symptoms all associated with one underlying problem.

Putting It All Together

So, what does the fire element have to do with hypothyroid? The thyroid is like the smoke alarm warning of fire and inflammation. As discussed, inflammation is an imbalance in the fire element. Inflammation, toxicity, and nutrient deficiency are often at the source or are the root cause of hypothyroidism and Hashimoto's disease (autoimmune thyroiditis). I often see high cholesterol levels in my hypothyroid patients, this is often due to the average American diet that is already shifting if you are following through with changes from the wood element.

Cleaning up our external environment also requires us to look at our relationships. Emotional stress from our heart space leads to further damage in an already out-of-balance system. How often have you seen lifelong partners pass away within months of each other? It's often said that the second partner gave up or died of a broken heart. Our connections with others either balance and fuel our drive and passion for life or drain us. The foggy brain can't remember why you went into a room, and drowsiness that accompanies hypothyroid symptoms is a function of the fire element. Think of a fire that had wet wood thrown on it; it's hard to light, creates a lot of smoke, and is generally slow to burn. When the liver or wood element is loaded down with toxins, it becomes sluggish and does not properly fuel the fire element.

Emotional-Body and Higher Self

The emotional aspects of the fire element are joy, passion, discernment, happiness, clarity, and mindfulness, and in combination with other elements, anxiety, rage, and sadness. A happy heart slows the pulse, calms the mind, and gives us clarity of discernment. A bitter heart is cold, fragile, and prone to blockage.

Love is often also associated with the heart in the Western world. As I mentioned earlier in Chapter 3, when speaking of language, there are many words for *love* in Chinese. And they do not distinguish love as an emotion per se or belonging to a particular element; it is just something that is present when all things are balanced. It is one of the highest vibrations of the human emotions and unconditional love is associated with the spiritual realm and higher Self in this case.

I often get asked "why (or how) are you always so happy?" And the truth is that I know that I am not always happy. But I have followed my intuition and gone toward things that brought me joy and away from situations that brought anger, frustration and feelings of being less or incapable for many years. I get sad, I get frustrated or even at times angry but can be with it and move forward because I've made a practice of noticing when those other emotions come up and dealing with them in a way the brings peace to me and the others involved. My anger these days generally stems from what seems like injustice in the world, some of which I can do something about and much that I can only live my life by example and hope that those that it will make a difference for learn to do the same. When I get sad or feel brokenhearted, it takes a little time sitting by the river of sorrow and letting my tears fill it up until I realize this is the same old "I'm not enough" in some way that has always been at the source of human suffering. If someone doesn't want to be with me or me with them doesn't mean anything is wrong. It just means that we're not a vibrational match to each other. And holding on to a situation like this causes more pain and sorrow. This is where we all have choice in acknowledging the emotion, the cause of it, and the mind-set behind it or choose suffering by being a victim to your experience. Where and how can you choose joy and compassion and send love from a distance to those who bring you the most suffering?

If you are looking for your passion or what brings you the most joy in life, I would say stop looking outside for something other than what you already know to be true for yourself. What are the things that when you do them the rest of the world fades away and you lose track of time? For me this was researching new and interesting things about spirituality and life and researching family history. Truth is, I love to learn new things and once I've satisfied my curiosity on a topic, I'm happy to move on. This makes me a Jack-of-many-trades sort of person. And mastery comes from "knowing thy Self." And then being thy Self!

When you create a circle of friends that you have amazing relatedness and conversation with, you know you are unconditionally loved. When you spend the majority of your time just being you in service to others and resting when needed, it's hard not to be happy, joyful, and at peace in your life. Comparing your outer circumstances to those around you kills joy, happiness, and connectedness with others.

Have you ever had that experience of connection with another person, where everything else falls away? In that moment, there is literally nothing there other than love and appreciation. Many people experience this when holding a newborn; looking into those magnificent little eyes, you feel your heart expand. No words are needed. This is the experience of a balanced fire element, where you are mind-body and heart connected; there is nothing to be discerned or released, as there is just pure, innocent love. There is a pull or a tug to want to stay in that experience and protect it for life. It's unfortunate that we are not able to treat all relationships with the same connectedness and love. Life experiences change all of us and the meaning we develop over time and the actions we take in reaction to those meanings are what make us "turbid," creating a need for discernment in relationships, our own actions, and who we want to be a part of our chosen family.

Familial relationships are often the most difficult relationships because we are tied to family members by blood. Our culture tells us that these are our people, yet, you likely have chosen a different path, left home, or just don't resonate with what family does. Your friends become your chosen confidants and they see you the most in the world outside your home. Friends are your chosen family or tribe. If you don't like what you see in the five people you see the most of, consider exploring activities you are passionate about and making new friends.

The gift of the fire element is compassion, empathy, and heart-centered communication.

Actions to Take

Environmental for Physical and Energetic

1. Turn of computers, TVs, and put down phones at least thirty minutes before bed.
2. Get a journal to brain dump in it before bed.

3. Spend five to ten minutes a day sitting quietly and focusing inward on your heart. I recommend a device called Muse – the brain sensing headband. It is an EEG biofeedback device that helps those learning to meditate to cue in to when you are in that state and when you are not. It is a great tool to use for meditation but is not required to get started!

Introspection for Mind and Emotional Bodies

1. Look at your relationships, starting with friendships, as they are easier to manage than family. As you think of the individual, do they fuel or drain you? Are you willing to spend less time with those who drain you, leaving you with more time to spend with those who fuel you?

2. What are you passionate about? If you don't know, give yourself permission to spend some time each week trying something you always wanted to.

3. Ask your body, "Are you moving enough?" Listen for the answer; if the answer is "yes," great. If the answer is "no," what type of movement does your body like? Exercise is often a foundational piece that is overlooked when we are busy and tired. Even a walk in the park or dancing around the living room or kitchen can shift the mood of the tired and sluggish.

4. We all have a warped sense of who we are and how other people see us. Ask five people you are close to what they see as your strengths and weaknesses, not from a place of judgment, but from a place of exploration and curiosity. You may be surprised by their answers.

CHAPTER 9

NOURISHMENT, FOOD SENSITIVITY, AND GROUNDING – THE EARTH ELEMENT

THE EARTH ELEMENT, MUCH LIKE OUR PLANET EARTH, IS THE foundation and center from which all the other elements flow and function. It is the soil, rock, and solid foundation for which we derive wellness. When we look to our environment for clues to our own well-being, we can see that healthy soil grows beautiful forests and plant life, while unhealthy soil leaves withered and diminished vegetation that is then eroded by winds and water.

Functional medicine practitioners view "the gut" as the foundation for healing most chronic health concerns. Without proper microbiome balance, the body continues to be in a state of inflammation. In Traditional Chinese Medicine the earth element is associated with the spleen and stomach.

Physical and Energetic Body

Unlike the anatomy and physiology books of Western medicine, the spleen is considered the most important organ in the digestive process and in creating Qi and blood. The blood we speak of here is not specifically the red stuff we seep when we cut our finger, but similar enough in nature that we can consider them one in the same. As we discussed earlier, Qi is the wave/particle, energetic being/ biochemical processing body that we are all made of. The spleen is responsible for governing the transportation and transformation, more specifically, the transformation of food into usable particles through the process of digestion and the transportation of those particles through the blood to where we need them to be – muscles, organs, brain, etc. The spleen is also given the responsibility of transportation and transformation of phlegm and fluids or water metabolism, which we can associate with the lymphatic system.

It is said that the spleen controls the blood and dominates the muscles and four limbs. It is this function that keeps the blood in the vessels, and when it is depleted, can seep blood, like bruising, heavy menstrual cycles, breakthrough bleeding, or hemorrhoids. The spleen is in charge of the muscles and adequate nutrition ensures well-developed muscles and control of the arms and legs.

The spleen opens into the mouth to give us a sense of taste and manifests on the lips. A rosy complexion and naturally pink lips are the sign of a healthy spleen, and the flavor associated with the earth element is sweet. Many people crave sweets, especially after eating a meal. This is the body's way of telling us that the spleen and stomach could use some support. The herbs that treat the earth element are sweet in nature but are *not* sugar. We actually weigh down the digestive process even more by adding a sugary dessert on top of a heavy meal that the body is already asking for support in processing. Because we are not taught about the five flavors in our culture, we automatically go to sugar when we crave sweet. Sugar and processed carbohydrates that generally accompany sugar cravings create "dampness," which is the way it feels when you eat too much; you feel bloated, full, and you may even wake up the next morning with swollen fingers on which your rings fit a little tight. Most people blame this on salt intake in our culture, but more often than not this is due to too much food and dampness of the earth element. A quick recap on the five flavors for each of the elements so far – wood was sour, fire was bitter, earth is sweet, the next two elements are metal and water, which are pungent and salty, respectively. The idea is not to feed your cravings but to notice them as a sign of imbalance and balancing the channels through diet and the other exercises of mind, energy, and spirit.

The partner to spleen (yin) is the stomach (yang), which dominates reception. If we are not receiving food to nourish our bodies, the spleen has nothing to work with. The stomach is said to receive, break down, and descend food into the body, where the spleen ascends it to the other organs. This yin/yang, up/down, opposition creates balance that if disrupted, can result in lack of appetite, vomiting, diarrhea, or the prolapse of organs.

Emotional Body

The emotions associated with the earth element are worry, will, self-nourishment (all yin – internal) and openness to receive (yang – external). When we think of the functions listed above from a spiritual context, the spleen is about processing life experiences and information, while the stomach is about receiving outer input – or a "gut feeling," as we often say. When we ignore our gut feeling or intuition in lieu of our brain or others telling us what we should do, we break the will of our Self and damage the energy of the spleen. There are so many expectations put on us by media, magazines, and what our mothers and teachers told us that we can't even hear what our own being needs. In our current society, we are so bombarded by information that has no valuable content that we often get caught up in all the noise and stop paying attention to what is important to our own Self and body. Much like our physical bodies are often overfed, although malnourished, so are our mind and spirit.

Is it any wonder that rates of ADD and ADHD in children have grown exponentially compared to what they were one hundred years ago? Children are so overstimulated by their environments and then handed little screens to entertain themselves, leading to further stimulating effects and little content value that they never learn to evaluate their own experiences and process them. It is normal and healthy to zone out for little while to process your life experiences. Children used to be brilliant at this; I can't tell you the number of times I watched my niece, sitting at the dinner table, zone out and be completely in her own little world long enough to process her experiences. Once her little three- to five-year-old brain made sense of things, she would rejoin us in conversation. This was the benefit of growing up in a rural area with little TV and screen time on enough land to run and play outside in nature.

Worry is an emotion that can literally be coded in our DNA. There is a particular gene that refers to the variations as the worrier or the warrior. This worry isn't necessarily about what everyone else thinks, although it can be, because we have all had the experience of feeling punched in the gut by someone else's word or opinion of us. Who doesn't want to avoid feeling that again? The warrior takes it as a challenge to fight back and the worrier sees it as an assault on their existence and worries what to do about, if they did the right thing, and what others think whether they did or did not. It is the worry of always looking to the future and creating all the possible things that could go wrong in the unknown and then second guessing their actions or words. Assaults to the energetic properties of our earth element feel like they rock your foundation or make you feel lower than dirt. Whether you are a worrier or a warrior, we have all experienced situations that put knots in our stomach or left us with nauseous feeling.

Years ago, I was part of a book group that discussed a book about archetypes that we all have. One of those archetypes was the victim. I hated the thought that we all had a victim archetype because I hated to admit that I had felt that way. I didn't want to face the part I played in being a victim. I didn't want to hear the words in my head that made me feel like I wasn't worthy over and over. And I didn't want to feel the pain of being spoken to or treated in a way that was so derogatory, and I didn't want to admit that on some level I believed the words and was shamed by the actions. When I uncovered that under all of my extra weight was a young girl and a young lady that had been devastated by the words of people who promised to love her until they died, I started to notice that I still, years later, made choices at every meal based on what I had come to believe… that I was born to be fat and I didn't deserve healthy food because it was more expensive and I didn't make as much money as someone else, I needed to eat less or what cost less. So, every visit to a restaurant, I looked for the cheapest meal or I chose a drive through with a dollar menu instead and every grocery store visit I bought the cheapest food or what was on sale. I had very little concept of what this was doing in my body at the time.

While my earthy foundation was strong, and I chose to leave the relationships that created that behavior and honor my own Self and self-expression, I had not let go of the damage that had been done emotionally. I know that over the generations, women were trained to serve their spouse and allowed their will to be set aside for the sake of the family unit. I see this in my clinic with my patients all the time; some people have no idea who they are without their defined rolls of mother, wife, sister, or employee. The past forty to fifty years have evolved the role of women in society, but we still struggle with identity in the world as individuals while in relationships. I work most often with women, but I also see similar patterns in men the more our culture evolves to become balanced within the individual instead of by others in relationship. There is no right answer for what you should do in your relationship situations. All I can say is be your Self. Stand for what and who you are, set boundaries and hold to them. If this is a continuous point of contention, then maybe it's not the best situation for you. When children are involved, it is understood that it is a much more complicated situation. And I have adult friends that will clearly admit that their parents getting a divorce was the best thing that happened for them to see the strength, beauty, and wisdom of their mother as she blossomed after the divorce. This doesn't mean it wasn't hard or that it was right or wrong and any other judgment. Just that the best things you can do for your children is to show them how to honor themselves by honoring your Self.

The Science and Medicine of the Earth Element

You are likely familiar with the anatomy of the body enough to know that the stomach is the little vessel filled with acid that our food dumps into once we swallow it. The stomach sits just below the diaphragm, where your ribs come up to attach to your sternum, directly above your navel. The stomach's functions are basically breaking down food before it delivers it to the small intestine.

The spleen, however, is less talked about and honestly even less understood in the science community. It is known to be the largest organ of the lymphatic system and has a role in the circulation of the immune system. The medical community knows that it stores platelets for clotting, white blood cells to fight bacterial infections, and recycles old red blood cells as the body replaces them. Beyond that, it is considered one of those organs you can live without if it were to be damaged.

The naturopathic community has long associated the spleen as having a role in leaky gut, which is a term that was not recognized by the medical community until recently with the growing functional medicine community. A recent study, titled "The spleen is the site where mast cells are induced in the development of food allergy," was published in the *Journal of International Immunology* in February 2017. It is only in the last few years that science has been able to actually show what is going on the development of all the sensitivities and allergies we hear about these days.

Leaky gut is a condition where, because of inflammation in the gut from unbalanced microflora, little gaps begin to form between the cells where usually the micronutrients we need to function and survive would be absorbed. As these little gaps appear, tiny food particles make it into the bloodstream, where they should not be. Our body's immune system tags these particles as dangerous and creates an immune response to them. This is how we create food sensitivities. Even minor gut imbalances that happen because of poor-quality food, pesticides, herbicides, and antibiotics can lead to leaky gut and food sensitivities over time. This is the biggest reason that cleaning up our diet by eating less processed food and more non-GMO and organic foods is more important than ever before.

Many people eat foods on a daily basis, unaware that they are sensitive to them. Allergies are pretty obvious in that their reaction occurs within thirty minutes of exposure and remains in the body for a couple of days. Sensitivities, on the other hand, can react anywhere from three hours to three days, making it nearly impossible to track the source without testing. I bring this up because many of my low-energy, sluggish, tired patients with dry skin and hair loss have food sensitivities to multiple foods. The biggest offenders that tend to make a huge difference when removed from the diet are wheat, corn, soy, dairy, and eggs.

As we discussed in Chapter 7, wheat is a high pesticide, GMO, herbicide offender, *and* it is often tagged by the immune system as harmful, creating sensitivities to it. Conventional corn is genetically modified to kill off certain bacteria and fungus. It does not stop that process once it is cut for consumption, therefore, in your gut it still kills off things that may be beneficial to your body, like healthy bacteria. Eating organic corn is a better choice. Soy has similar issues as well as being a hormone disruptor. When grown organically and fermented like it was traditionally used in Asian cultures, it can be highly beneficial.

Some may say gluten-free or food-elimination diets are fads, but the reality is there to support that in the United States our genetic modifications and farming practices have turned wheat, corn, and soy into products where the cost of inflammation outweighs the benefit to our bodies. And it is often just best to eliminate these foods.

There are many types of food allergy testing out there. Some of the best I have worked with look at not only the IgE (actual allergy, reacts in thirty minutes) and IgG (sensitivity, can have reaction three to seventy-two hours later) but also other components of the immune system, like IgG4 (which is protective against IgE, but without IgE response is a sensitivity) and C3d (which ramps up the response to the IgG sensitivity). If your practitioner is only looking at only IgG or IgE from a blood sample or a whelp from old-school scratch testing on your skin, they are likely missing the overall picture of your responses to foods. By knowing what you are responding negatively to, you can cut these out for a period of time while using collagen, aloe, and glutamine to heal the gut, and pre- and probiotics to replenish and balance. For some it takes more than these, and it is recommended to work with a functional medicine practitioner. By taking these actions I have been able to start eating some organic foods again that used to make my mouth itch and give me severe heartburn. Other foods, like wheat, I have found I am just happier and healthier without and rarely miss. Once I started feeling much better by cutting out the foods on my allergy and sensitivity list, I was able to tell when I put them back in how bad I felt when eating them and the weird symptoms they triggered, like rosacea and acne that had nothing to do with why I ran allergies in the first place.

I learned which foods made me feel tired, sluggish, constipated, or foggy brained. Within the first few weeks of cutting out these foods most people notice their clothes being looser, especially around the waist, as well as more energy and fewer symptoms overall. The number on the scale, however, doesn't always change. I had one patient drop two pant sizes in the waist in two weeks by getting rid of the foods causing the inflammation in the gut and it only changed the scale about five pounds. I'm not saying that everyone's hypothyroid symptoms are allergy and sensitivity based. I am saying that it is worth looking into if bloating in your middle or other digestive issues are also part of your symptoms.

Mind-Body

The mind-body in the earth element is about overthinking and learning to be mindful and present while eating. In wood, we worked with ego and visualizing; the fire element is about heart-centered communication, and now, in earth, we have to get grounded. Without getting grounded, you tend to spend too much time in your head planning and ruminating on what has come before or what is to come. Grounding helps us bring into alignment our mental, energetic, and physical bodies, which in turn calms the emotional body. When we are in our heads overthinking, it consumes calories, but it does not differentiate what you are getting those calories from. This is the "snack and think" phenomena of mindless eating that so many of us did as college students. This is why many coaches tell you to turn off the TV and distractions when eating as a way to measure your fullness, react to what you are eating, and know what you like and don't like that you stuff in your face.

Did you even taste your food? There are many times in life when I overscheduled myself and ended up eating whatever I could find in ten minutes – sometimes in the car on the way to somewhere. This is not a healthy habit, no matter your age. Honestly, I can't even remember tasting my food; I'm not sure I liked it, but it filled the space in my stomach. When I am grounded and intentional, I don't overschedule, forget to bring my own food, overeat, or overindulge for reward. When you are mindful while eating, grounded, and present in your physical body, you will start to notice that food you thought was your favorite doesn't taste that good anymore. You may have even made up your mind that you loved that particular meal as a seven-year-old. For me, this was Cheetos. Don't get me wrong, the memory centers in my brain still think crunchy, salty, and cheesy would be good but then the fact that they disintegrate into that weird-tasting paste after being chewed is now kind of gross to me. And I've always loved Mexican food; however, the more mindful I am when I eat, the less of it I actually want, and what I choose to eat is different at Mexican restaurants.

So how do you get grounded? There are all sorts of ways. Visualizing growing roots from your feet into the earth, taking a walk barefoot in the grass, hugging a tree, or repotting a plant are great ways to ground yourself. Get your hands in the dirt, wiggle your toes into the sand at the beach, or even just put focus on feeling your toes, calves, thighs, and similar, in the moment. Many people find that exercising in nature is particularly grounding. YouTube also has many grounding meditations to follow along if you prefer having a guiding voice.

Higher Self

This is the one element where accessing your higher Self comes through getting grounded and in touch with the physical body. Observe what you notice about your gut reactions to food, life, people, and so on, not from a place of thinking, but from a place of just taking note. When I first started eating and cooking clean,

I would sit down to eat and notice this little tingle of excitement, almost like a baby wiggling her toes when she takes the first few bites of a food she loves. Additionally, the foods I ate were not choices I would have made for the "old" me.

Actions to Take

Environmental for Physical and Energetic

1. After clearing out the foods mentioned in the wood element chapter (Chapter 7), if you are still having digestive problems, consider working with a functional medicine practitioner to learn about your food allergies and sensitivities.

2. Probiotics can be a great addition to a daily regimen, but they are not all equal, and depending on your body, there are likely strains that are more beneficial than others. Yogurt does not count here. It does not have enough live strains, is often filled with sugar, and whatever live strains are there often get killed off in the stomach before it ever makes it to the intestines where it is needed. If you have been taking the same probiotic for a long time, it is a good idea to switch it up, as too much of a good thing is no longer beneficial and can lead to further imbalance.

3. Boost your immune system by cleaning up your diet and starting a regular exercise routine. If that part is hard for you, hire a trainer to help keep you accountable.

4. Get grounded with the exercises mentioned above or in whatever way gets you present to your physical body in the here and now.

Introspection for Mind and Emotional Bodies

1. Are you a worrier? If yes, notice how often you worry about things that you have no control over. Think of one of those worries. Write it down. What are the actual facts about the here and now? (Write them down). What are the feelings in your body around those facts? Notice what your thoughts about it are versus what you feel. Write that down. Now write down the worst things that could happen, and ask if that is true right now? Now ask yourself if that happens, what can you do about it? It will look something like:
   ○ I'm worried about publishing what I've written.
   ○ The facts are I've spent time and money to go to school, work in my field for years, write a book, and get it edited, and it's almost done.
   ○ I feel a sinking in my gut and fear of potential criticism or getting in trouble somehow.
   ○ Worst case scenario, someone writes a bad review.
   ○ The fear is real, the sinking in my gut is real, but it is not true now and may never be.
   ○ If it happens, I will deal with it then. Because right now there is nothing I can do about it.
   ○ Often what we notice is that our emotions are very real in the moment but solicited by something that may never come to be. The key is catching yourself in worry and breaking it down in the moment before it overwhelms you.
2. Notice where you break your own will. Do you say you are going to work out three times this week and then find reasons not to or just stay in bed and blow it off? Do you say you are going to be more social and then turn down invitations to do so? Strengthening your own resolve strengthens your earth element.

CHAPTER 10

BREATHE AND LET GO – THE METAL (AIR) ELEMENT

METAL MAY SEEM OUT OF PLACE IN THE FIVE ELEMENTS, AND it is often referred to as air in the traditional medicines of Native American, Ayurvedic, and other cultures. While it absolutely has to do with air as well, it is called metal for the properties and taste it correlates with. Metal is strong; it is often used for its durability, strength, and malleability. It was used throughout time to create tools and armor, and rarer, softer metals are used for jewelry. Metal itself comes from primary elements on the periodic chart of elements, and it is as much a part of our planet as water, fire, and wood.

Physical and Energetic Body

In traditional Chinese medicine, the element of metal is associated with the lung and large intestine. You may think this is an odd combination, but have you ever noticed that when you get a sinus infection, it is often accompanied by constipation? Which came first is a bit like the chicken and the egg, but the two often occur together. The responsibility of the lung is to dominate the Qi, disperse it downward, maintain the skin and hair, and regulate the passage of water. The large intestine absorbs fluid and let go of waste. The metal element opens to the nose, giving us a sense of smell; relates to the emotion of grief; and when imbalanced is associated with a metallic taste in the mouth.

When we breathe in, Qi (the air particles, oxygen, and energetic essence of the world around us) comes from the exterior to the interior. This is the only internal organ of the body that is allowed to mingle with the outside world. Ideally, we inhale pure, clean air and exhale CO_2 and other "waste Qi." It is said that inhalation or the act of inspiration is "the Qi of heaven being in communication with the lung." The original roots of the words *respiration*, *expiration*, and *inspiration* are all one in the same. When we breathe in, it is to bring in the Qi of heaven (inspiration); when we exhale (expiration), we breathe out that which no longer served us or was pathogenic; and when we do that over and over (respiration). As languages and meaning change over time, we came to think of inspiration as divine thought dropping into our consciousness, expiration as death, and respiration as breathing.

Breathing greatly influences the functional activities of the whole body. When we don't breathe properly, we can either have a lack of oxygen that leads to lassitude, sluggishness, or shortness of breath. On the other hand, if we breathe too deeply, we can become light-headed and hyperventilate or hyper-oxygenate the tissues, leaving a tingling sensation.

Skin and hair are regulated by the element of metal. Skin is our protective armor that is also porous and allows entrance and exit of what we come in contact with. As hunter-gatherers, this gave us exposure to essential oils from the plants we worked around, walked on, and harvested. Our sweat releases toxins and excess minerals back to the earth and acts as a cooling system. These days, unless we purposely put essential oils on our skin, we do not come into contact with native plants in our area. If we walk barefoot in the grass, we are likely absorbing pesticides, herbicides, and chemical fallout from the air and fertilizer.

Wei Qi, or Protective Qi, is the part of the immune system that protects us from external pathogens, such as viruses and unhealthy bacteria. When our lungs are strong and functioning properly and our large intestine eliminates properly, our Wei Qi is strong. When our metal element functions are weak, there is a hole in our armor that allows in pathogens. To improve this function, practice the breathing exercise at the end of this chapter.

The function of the large intestine is to absorb the water from the waste that was brought to it by the small intestine after being processed by the functions of the spleen and stomach and the nutrients already absorbed into the system. Bowel movements can be indicators of health. At first, many of my patients don't like to talk about their bathroom habits but, over time, become accustomed to me asking. We all poop (I think this might be the title of a children's book), and consistency, color, and odor can give insight into dysfunction. Constipation, which is often associated with hypothyroid, is when waste material sits in the large intestine too long; more waste material is compacted together with either not enough water to trigger the movement of it or not enough movement and too much water being absorbed.

Getting moving, even a thirty-minute walk a day, can remedy the latter, while drinking enough water to support your body's clearance of waste material is also important. A general rule of thumb is to drink approximately half your weight in ounces of water a day. Preferably, drink room temperature or warm water, as it takes less energy to warm it up than ice water. For most people, drinking enough water means four to six ounces of water an hour in your sixteen waking hours. Dumping thirty-two ounces in your system in a twenty-minute-window is not as useful as four to eight ounces consumed four to eight times a day. The body cannot absorb all of it at once, and it flushes straight through to the kidneys and bladder, without serving the purpose we drank it for in the first place. Other cultures do not drink so much water with food, as we do in the United States. Instead, other cultures reserve drinking water for outside of mealtime. This lets the stomach do its job of breaking down foods without watering down the contents in the stomach.

The taste of the metal element is pungent. The herbs that treat it are pungent and include such as foods like onion, garlic, ginger, radishes, and mustard.

Emotional Body

Grief sticks with us like a wound in our soul that just won't heal. Time does make it better, but there is still a soreness – a sadness – to the wound that is touched again and again by memories, reminders, and the on-coming grief of others. Once you have lost someone close to you, whether it was an unborn child, a parent, a partner, or a child, the devastating emotional impact temporarily affects the immune system and leaves you open to catching the viral cold going around or flare-ups of old viruses that hide out in your body. Grief is not limited to the loss of loved ones but also includes the loss of potential futures that comes about because of break ups, divorce, or even failed business ventures. This grief may be less severe than the death of a loved one, but it is still grief none the less.

Many years ago, I had a patient come in with a persistent cough that was made worse by cleaning chemicals. We talked about ways to clean with healthier products, and she shifted this in her home and her new job. We worked on typical seasonal allergies, but the cough persisted. One day, I asked her about grief. She smiled, as tears welled up in her eyes, and she explained that a few years before, she created a humanitarian project that progressed well until her previous boss found out. He gave her the option of shutting it down or losing her job, as it seemed a conflict of interest to him. She was devastated but couldn't support herself or her project without a job. As this was not a typical loss of life, no one in her circle of support understood her grief, so she left it unprocessed. By giving witness to her grief, lessening her chemical load, and balancing the other elements of stress in her life, she stopped coughing and began to feel stronger.

For some, this theory of "stuck emotions" seems "woo woo," weird, or irrelevant, as it seems to have little to do with the physical body. I'm not saying that emotions are the problem; rather, I'm saying that the energetic wave of emotion, when stopped, may manifest as a physical symptom that can be released by observing its presence in the subconscious and physical. It relates back to the wave particle theory and the integration of the physical, emotional, and mind-bodies. Let me also be clear that I'm not saying it is all in your head, that you have control, or that it is your fault. These sorts of things are no one's fault; we didn't attract the experience and it is definitely not a thought problem. It's like having a piece of rubber dragging underneath your car that throws debris and sparks. Others around you can see it, but you can't. It just feels like something is not quite right. Others around you may point at it, honk their horn (talk about it), even motion you over (tell you about it), but you have no idea what their problem is with you. Well, they don't have a problem with you, specifically; they are just pointing to what could be dangerous to you, your health, and the ones around you. Slow down and take a look for yourself. Are there unprocessed emotions just under the surface that are ready to be released? If so, acknowledge them, breathe, and let go! If it seems too much, visualize handing them over to God, Source, or whatever higher power you believe in.

Mind-Body

In the element of metal (air) there can also be patterns of lacking inspiration, not letting go, and holding on to beliefs that no longer serve you. As small children, we are all programmed to the beliefs in our community, country, and home. If this is all you know, then it is just the way it is, much like when people believed the world was flat. This sort of belief does not make us sick. It is just something that we don't know we don't know, and until we start to explore it, there is nothing more. Introspection and exploration help point to areas where we could have more freedom and self-expression. Freedom to be self-expressed and surrounded by others that support us, just as we are, helps build a healthy sense of well-being, not necessarily health. A lack of inspiration can leave you feeling stagnant and stuck, repeating the same patterns day after day, not knowing what else to do or even why you were doing it in the first place.

There is a story about an old monk in a temple who was leading meditation. There had been a litter of kittens born on the grounds and one of the kittens had come to join them for meditation. The kitten began to meow and howl, making the most awful noises. The monk asked one of the others to take the kitten to a room and close it up so that it wasn't a disturbance for those meditating. The next day at meditation time, the kitten came back, repeated the scenario, and was locked up. For the next twenty years, before meditation started, they took the cat to the back room and locked it up. The old monk passed away and the cat was becoming slow and elderly as well, and one day passed away. The monks who had been there for fifteen years or more went out to find another cat to lock up in the same room. They never stopped to consider why; it was just what was done for meditation time.

I tell this story here to remind us to evaluate how we spend some of our precious time repeating things that no longer serve us. For me, this habit was coming home, sitting down on the couch, and playing games on my phone for hours on end and feeling like I just didn't have the time to get everything done. At one point in time, this gave me an outlet to keep my mind sharp while my body rested and recovered. It gave me the satisfaction of a win when the financial and emotional world around me all felt like losses. At some point, I came to the realization that the games on my phone and tablet were no longer enough to keep me entertained; I continued to play them and have the TV on while I was on the computer. All the distraction still wasn't enough to stop the sadness of loss of my father, grandparents, relationships, and sense of freedom. I felt stuck and had no idea what to do next. However, I kept myself so busy that I didn't think I had time to do anything else. It wasn't until I turned the devices off, set them aside, and started to feel that I found some other outlets of things I enjoyed. I began to cook foods I didn't even know I loved, interact with more people in my world, and go for walks outside.

The Science and Medicine of the Metal Element

Chronic feelings of fatigue have recently been associated with reactivation of Epstein-Barr Virus (EBV) or human herpesvirus (HHV); there are more than two hundred studies on PubMed.gov (an online resource for published biomedical articles) connecting the two. I'm not saying you have EBV or HHV, but if you have never been tested, it might be worth looking into. As mentioned earlier in this chapter, when there is imbalance in the lung, large intestine, or our immune system because of the stressors of grief, unclean air, and poor breathing habits, we are more likely to get or flare up an old viral infection.

When looking at breathing on pubmed.gov, I found are over 327,000 articles, 9,800 of which are associated with breathing exercises. To say that breathing is important is an understatement; it is literally one of the components our life depends on. Breathing alone can help reduce stress, increase energy and digestion, lower blood pressure, reduce sleepiness during the day, improve sleep quality at night, increase fertility, and so much more.

Higher Self

As indications of our higher Self, we can let our physical symptoms guide us where to look for information. If you have no digestive or lung issues, that's awesome. However, many patients have already been diagnosed with IBS, colitis, Crohn's, diverticulitis, or some other version of inflammation or perforation in the large intestine.

Depending on which version you were diagnosed with, it might go something like this – the large intestine is where we absorb the last remnants of our nourishment. If you are irritated by that nourishment, you may have developed sores, or it may have eaten away at you for a while. What are some of those experiences that should have nourished you but turned out to be traumatic? It may be one of those childhood stories again. For me, it started as always being an overachiever in school, always feeling like I was expected to be the best and competitive enough that I wanted to be the best. One day, I came home with my report card, proud of my ninety-six in precalculus, and my father looked at it, smiled, and said, "Only a ninety-six in math? Had you stayed off the phone and studied, you would have gotten a one hundred."

I was devastated; my grade was the best grade in the class, and I don't think study time had anything to do with my grade not being perfect. However, it perpetuated my already unhealthy drive of perfectionism. This stuck with me until I revisited it in my early thirties, could see my father just wanted what was best for me, and let it go. I couldn't be perfect or even the best all the time – actually, most of the time. Someone was always going to have learned more on a particular topic, or be faster, stronger, or better paid for the same or less work. While this partially is mind and emotional body associated, emotionally shutting down my pride and energetically pulling back in my energy that had been beaming, my body began to be more stagnant. These are not issues that started in my thirties when I dealt with hypothyroid concerns. Instead, incidences like this build up over time. The more rigid we become, the more severe our experiences are, and the more we compare ourselves with others kills our progression to be our best Self.

The gift of the metal element is expanded feeling (touch). This is the energetic sensitive that can feel textures of emotion (empath) or dysfunction when running their hand near another's body (kinesthetic).

When we breathe in inspiration and let go of all the negativity we've been holding on to emotionally and energetically, our higher Self soars and guides us clearly.

Action Item: Breathing Exercise

To improve circulation of Qi and strengthen your lung capacity try this exercise. With your tongue lightly touching the roof of your mouth, visualize breathing in a ball of white light (pure, clear energy) through your nose, down your throat, behind your sternum, through the diaphragm, and all the way below your umbilicus. Breathe out, pushing that white ball of energy down between your legs, wrapping it around to your spine, and climbing back up over the top of your head and out your nose. Continue this breathing pattern for ten minutes, noticing where you feel like you lose your breath or feel pain or stuckness. As you feel those areas, focus on the next round, pushing the ball of light through that area to complete the circle. At first, many people notice that they don't breathe below their diaphragm. If you watch babies breathe, their abdomen rises and falls more than their chest. As adults, we start holding in our gut and barely breathing. Reestablishing deep, belly breathing increases circulation, calms the mind and heart rate, and decreases blood pressure and pain.

CHAPTER 11

DRINK MORE AND CLEANSING RITUALS – THE WATER ELEMENT

WATER IS SUCH AN INTEGRAL PART OF OUR PLANET (71 percent), our bodies (average 70 percent water), and everything that makes Earth hospitable for life. Water carves away at the earth, making majestic canyons and layering the sediment back into the depths of the ocean where it will one day rise and become mountains again. Much like the mysterious depths of unexplored oceans, the water element holds many secrets to life.

The Physical Body

The organs associated with the water element are kidney and urinary bladder. The kidney, unlike the previous organs, has distinctly yin and yang functions, as well as essence and kidney Qi functions.

In general, the kidney is responsible for storing essence and dominating development and reproduction. This refers to our own life stages of puberty and menopause in women, as well as the actual creation of fetus and birth. Essence, in this sense, refers to the material base of the human body and its functional activities. While there is much more to this essence than just DNA, it can be associated with the genetic material we get from our parents (congenital essence) and the materials used from foods we bring into our bodies (acquired essence). While we can't change our congenital essence (DNA and birth story) because it was what we were born with, we can absolutely change our acquired essence by what we choose to eat. These foundational components of essence are absolutely at the source of our health and well-being.

The kidney dominates water metabolism as an activity of Qi and separates the clear and turbid. The turbid water, or dirty water, is then stored in the urinary bladder until it is excreted. Dysfunction of this process can lead to edema, retained fluids, and excess weight due to water retention. Often, the extra ten pounds put on by the hypothyroid patient is due to water weight. In conjunction with the spleen's transformation and transportation of fluids we discussed in Chapter 9, the kidney energy is also key in relieving some of the excess weight and puffiness.

Kidney has the functions of receiving Qi. Earlier, we discussed that the lung is responsible for breathing in Qi and dispersing it throughout the body. Well, the kidney grasps onto it and pulls it downward. Dysfunction of the kidney Qi can lead to shortness of breath or difficulty taking a deep breath, and this grasp of kidney Qi is in part associated with fertility. Taking deep breaths, down into the area of the womb, energizes our reproductive cycles. Low libido can be a result of breathing shallowly or not grasping onto breath.

Kidney also dominates the bone, manufactures marrow to fill up the brain, opens to the ears, and manifests in the hair. Here, the spinal cord and brain are referred to as the sea of marrow. Foggy brain and hair loss symptoms in hypothyroidism are a dysfunction of the kidney energy. As we age, the depletion of this kidney energy can lead to weaker bones and hearing loss.

Kidney yin is the foundation of yin fluid in the body, and it moistens and nourishes the other organs, muscles, tendons, skin, and hair. When yin fluid is not being moved properly by Qi, it results in dry skin, lack of hair luster or hair loss, and achy joints.

Kidney yang is responsible for balancing kidney yin by warming the body and promoting movement. A lack of kidney yang shows up as low energy, coldness, pain, or achiness in the lower back and knees and an aversion to cold and infertility. There are other reasons these symptoms could show up, but these are the tale tell signs of kidney yang deficiency. The best ways to nourish kidney yang are by following the guidelines for cleaning up your diet (Chapter 7), reducing anxiety and stress, getting enough sleep (Chapter 8), eliminating foods that create inflammation (Chapter 9), eliminating properly (Chapter 10) and releasing fears and lack.

Menopause and lessening of seminal fluid in men that happens after the age of fifty is the kidney's way of preserving congenital Qi and essence. By redirecting the use of kidney essence, Qi, and yin and yang to body functions instead of reproduction, it extends our life potential.

Last but not least, the kidney is responsible for the health of bones and teeth, and the associated taste is salty. So, if you are a crunchy/salty craver, this is a sign that your kidney energy needs support. In nature, carnivorous animals chew on bones for the crunchy/salty nourishment of calcium and the nutrients in bone marrow. This is one of the reasons that bone broth has become one of the crazes of the holistic community in recent years. Bone broth is a great nutrient for rebuilding gut, supporting bone and marrow strength, and healing the tissues of the body as well as kidney energy. Salty cravings can also be an indicator of adrenal stress.

Mind-Body

As the deepest of the elements, the mind-set piece is more about introspection and diving deep to discover the limiting beliefs and fears we all have, going inward to look at what is working and not working in our lives. Once you have a clear picture of what you want more of and what you need to let go of, it gives you the opportunity to create something new. This is one area where you have more answers for yourself than any book can give you. Try setting a plan for the next three months, it takes at least that long to really experience what something would be like as a lifestyle. What are things you think you should be doing? How often? And then commit to trying it out. You may find it is a perfect fit for your lifestyle and choose to continue doing it once the three months is over. You may also discover that you can hardly wait to quit what you committed to because it just doesn't work for your life, but don't quit before the three months is up! What you discover about yourself by doing something that isn't a fit for your lifestyle for three months is just as valuable as what you discover does work. An example would be: I think I should go to the gym to exercise at least thirty minutes five times a week. Commit to yourself and someone you trust to keep you accountable to do just that. Put something at stake, if you don't follow through, you owe them dinner or twenty dollars or something of value to you. (It is even fun to have them set their own accountability to you, if they are up for it – you can't push them into something and expect them to follow through; it won't work.) Check in throughout the week that you did what you said you would do. At the end of three months readjust the length of time or how many times or some of the specifics and keep going. I recommend creating these sort of experiences around numerous areas of your life: exercise and fitness, eating, relationship building (quality time with husband, children, and others), alone time for pampering yourself or experiencing something new, meditation, and so on. What many people find is that some things they thought they should do are just not a fit for them, some things made a huge difference and others were enjoyable but not so much helpful.

More importantly, it tests how committed you are to making a difference for yourself and your integrity around doing so.

Emotional Body

The emotion associated with the water element is fear. Is it any surprise that children with nightmares wet the bed or that our aging population has an increasing need for bladder control? Things that we did not fear in our younger years become scarier to many of our elders, such as the reality of pain or lack of mobility from breaking bones, loss of senses, such as hearing and memory, and the unknown of what comes next.

Fear is not only an emotion of children and the elderly, but it lurks in the periphery of our consciousness every day. Fear of getting hurt (emotionally) or being judged keeps us from saying what is real for us. Fear of failing keeps us from pursuing our dreams and taking chances in business. Fear of the opinions of others leads us to stuff our emotions and not live our fully self-expressed lives. As we have spoken of earlier, in the five elements, those stuffed emotions and lack of self-expression tend to dampen the functioning of our overall system.

When faced with something new, many people have a sense of fear — a fear of the unknown. For some, the feeling of excitement is so close to their fear of the unknown that they want to fight against new, exciting prospects in life because they don't already know the outcome. This type of fear experience leaves you stuck and in the same place and process, year after year, until something traumatic forces you to move.

Facing fear in micro-doses intentionally helps to move past fear responses in bigger situations. Walking the mini ropes course in the arcade with my niece or rock climbing with my nephew are ways that I face my fear of heights that has grown as I aged. Everyone's fears are different, so I'm not saying that everyone should go rock climbing if you've never been. That may be something you wanted to do but were afraid to. If so, try it in a gym that has proper gear and supervision. The idea here is to notice when your fear stops you. If there is something active that you always wanted to do, try it. The simple act of facing a fear in an environment where you are completely supported will help you move forward in other areas of your life. The sense of accomplishment of facing your fears leaves you energized and gives you a boost to go after other areas where fear has stopped you.

Energetic Body

Much like anger is expansive energetically, fear contracts. We've all heard some version of "she's just a wall flower" or "wow, her energy just fills the room when she walks in!" This is how we perceive another person's energy. Expansion and contraction of energy is normal, like breathing, but when it is out of balance for extended periods because of the same emotion, it becomes unhealthy. With fear, the tension that keeps the body in a state of contraction limits the flow of energy throughout the body and in turn reduces blood flow and life-giving nutrients. Practicing facing your fears, understanding the source of your anger, creating healthy relationships based in love and compassion, acknowledging and moving past worry, and letting go of grief, all help to move the energy associated with emotions which in turn moves the energy associated with the physical body.

Higher Self

In the language of the mind, water has to do with life experiences. Being able to sort out (wood) and absorb those life experiences (metal) without all of the turbid mind chatter (fire) and input from our relationships (earth), is the invaluable communication of messages between body and spirit. When you take time to sit and reflect on your daily experiences and not making someone else's action mean anything about you, you are able to be in relationships without fear. This way, you are capable of letting go and recreating with ease as needed.

Science and Medicine of the Thyroid and Adrenals

In TCM, there is no specific organ that relates to the functioning of the thyroid, adrenals, or other glands. I tend to think of them as adjuncts to the water and earth elements. The adrenal glands are closely linked with the kidneys, as they sit right on top of them, just under your ribs and below your scapulae. The adrenals are regulated by the hypothalamus and pituitary. Remember when we spoke of fight or flight response and the HPA axis? This is where it fits in. We are triggered by fear, most likely subconscious fear, to produce signals from the brain to trigger release of epinephrine (a.k.a. adrenalin). As the system is flooded with epinephrine, it feeds back to the hypothalamus, which sends message to the pituitary to send out cortisol (a steroid), which sends a message to the adrenals to produce norepinephrine (nor-adrenalin) to counteract the release of epinephrine so that our bodies can go back to rest, digest, and reproduce. When we are consistently bombarded with adrenalin-producing activities – driving a car; dealing with deadlines and bosses; listening to news of war, pandemic viruses, and murder; watching action T.V.; hearing loud, startling noises; and so much more – our bodies overproduce these neurochemicals to the point of exhaustion and confusion. The thyroid is also part of this system, as it is also regulated by the hypothalamus and pituitary.

Actions to Support Water Element

Drink More Water

Drink plain, clear water, preferably purified and not stored in plastics. As a general rule, consume half of your weight in ounces. However, as we discussed, do not drink it all at once. We are not camels and cannot store the thirty-two ounces of water you waited to drink until bedtime. Additionally, this does not support healthy sleep patterns because drinking so much fluid before bed is likely to wake you up in the night to go to the bathroom.

Put a glass or stainless-steel cup at your desk and set a reminder on your phone if necessary to get you to drink four to six ounces every hour throughout the day. Coffee, tea, and sodas do *not* count. While they may be wet, they are acidic and often dehydrating, so the body must spend more energy to separate the components out from the water.

Be Mindful of Sodium Intake

Salt, in its pure form, is not bad for us in moderate quantities. In fact, we need sodium and chloride in our bodies as electrolytes for certain functions. Salt, as it comes out of the earth, has a variety of trace minerals your body needs for proper functioning. Salt was originally considered a valuable preservative and was even used as currency. Over time, salt became a preferred taste and was changed to being listed as a flavoring. While we absolutely need salt, there is generally enough naturally occurring sodium in meats and vegetables to provide our sodium need.

In 1924, iodized salt became table salt to help the general population get the iodine needed to support the thyroid and reduce the quantity of goiters. Recently, in the healthy cooking circles, table salt or iodized salt has been set aside in favor of going back to sea salt or pink Himalayan salt. Therefore, getting iodine from natural sources, like kelp, seaweed, dulce, and similar, has become important to support your thyroid. When you consume too much salt, which processed foods are loaded with, you risk storing extra water in your body, which can cause high blood pressure and kidney stones, and can put stress on your heart, blood vessels, and brain, as well as cause swelling in your hands, feet, and other tissues throughout the body.

CHAPTER 12

.... -•-◇-•- ....

THE ELEMENTS: FLOW AND DESTRUCTION

NOW THAT WE HAVE TAKEN A DEEP DIVE INTO THE individual elements, it is important to see how they relate to each other. The ancient teachings of TCM listed the elements in directions with earth at the center, as we spoke of in Chapter 9, with water in the North, fire in the South, metal in the West, and wood in the East. The assumption was made that fire and water were true yang and yin and that wood and metal (air) were transition states, as they both had characteristics of the other elements. Over time, as the system evolved and our knowledge and understanding of it grew, earth was moved out in the circle with the other elements with the understanding that both yin and yang are present in all elements.

Now, each of the elements feed and flow into the next. Wood fuels fire, which nourishes earth, creating metal, that in turn enriches water, which feeds wood. When we are balanced in this cycle, it will occur like this: our personal growth (wood) brings us joy (fire), which nourishes our will (earth), so that we can let go of what no longer serves us (metal), and re-create (water) our vision (wood) filled with passion (fire), which nourishes our physical body (earth). Then, we walk right through our fear (water) to continue growing (wood) healthy relationships (fire), which build our confidence (earth), so we can breathe easier (metal) even in the grief of losing those in our life (water), as death is a part of life.

The flow of the physical body is a process of detoxing our system (wood), cooling the inflammation (fire), while feeding our bodies clean nourishing foods (earth), helping to let go of waste (metal), and drinking plenty of water to wash away and eliminate toxicity.

In the emotional body, we notice our frustration (wood) with our health and our lack of passion for life (fire). We worry about what is wrong (earth), grieve the losses in our lives (metal), and fear (water) what is to come if it doesn't get better. This is a normal process that points us to looking inward and making changes in our lives. If our anger (wood) over not making progress when eating healthy causes us to binge eat junk food (earth), we don't eliminate toxins properly (metal) and become puffy and swollen (water).

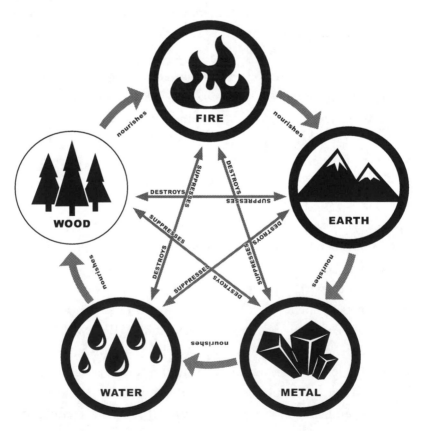

When the elements are weak, hyperactive, or just used out of order, the cycle becomes destructive or suppressive. Notice how we skipped over the community/joy aspect of the fire element in the last example. This, in turn, caused a burden on the earth element, which then skipped the proper functioning of metal, and overtaxed our ability to rid the body of water. Long-term dysfunction like this can cause high blood pressure because there's too much water in the system, which congests our blood vessels and heart (fire).

The destructive cycle skips over the next element and attacks the following one – fire melts metal (or sucks the oxygen from the air), metal chops wood, wood depletes the earth or replaces it with roots, and earth fills in or muddies the water, which puts out the fire. The suppressive cycle suggests that fire suppresses water by turning it into steam, water moves earth and forges canyons and mudslides, earthquakes uproot trees, and wood dulls metal.

How this shows up in everyday life could be as simple as swallowing your angry words (suppressed wood) and ending up with a sore throat (metal) or sinus congestion. Perhaps you had a huge fight (too much wood) with your loved one and ended up with an upset stomach (wood skips fire and destroys earth). On the other hand, maybe your stomach's upset because you ate too many rich, fatty foods (earth) that suppressed your liver and gall bladder (wood).

Usually, these incidents don't involve the whole system – not everything is destroyed at once. However, over time, wearing down the cycle can contribute to long-term health problems (chronic disease) and dysfunction. Remember how I always had respiratory allergies making the metal element weaker? Antibiotics further unbalanced my digestive system (earth) that then could no longer support nourishing the metal element (lung and large intestine). Inflammation (fire) continued to build, as it had nowhere to go but to further attack the metal element, which was already weakened.

Until I took herbs that helped clear the fire and support the earth, my breathing continued to worsen. Most people can start to follow their own progression of disease after reading through the processes I have given, but we often still need to do lab testing to sort out what nutrients are needed and to make sure nothing else is lurking beneath the surface, unbalanced.

You are capable of making the lifestyle changes previously mentioned that help you feel more energetic and alive while living a healthier life and teaching your children to make better choices than the generations before us. Taking this journey one step at a time and listening to your body about what does and doesn't work for you is your best ally. Each step toward a cleaner and healthier lifestyle is a step in the right direction. Celebrate yourself at each step and honor your body and your process.

I often get asked, "When do you stop trying to do it yourself or with alternative medicine and see an MD?" My answer is often that seeing your primary care physician regularly is always a good idea so you can have an established relationship for when, or if, you do need them. However, you always have the right to educate yourself, to choose to follow or not to follow an MD's recommendation, and/or to get another opinion.

Remember the phases from Chapter 4, leading from optimal, stressed, adapted, fatigued and functional to physiological then death? Nutrition (food as well as supplementation) is important at every stage, all the way up to the death process. There isn't much that can be done in the way of food when someone is catastrophically ill. Stress reduction and lifestyle (meditating, sleeping, dancing, laughing, getting a massage, and enjoying nature and good company) are great at every stage. Essential oils can be amazing for stress reduction and can change your mood, anchor mind-set changes, and improve cellular function. Acupuncture, Ayurveda, homeopathic remedies, naturopathy, and chiropractic practices are all good ways to improve from the stressed phase all the way to the physical manifestation. Herbs and supplements are great to reverse adaptation through physical complaints. Of course, functional medicine is doing an amazing job turning around health for the fatigued to physical gap between mostly holistic and lifestyle intervention to true medical necessity.

I realize the majority of my readers are not experts in any of these modalities and that is why we are here to help in whatever way we can and if we can't, point you in the direction of others who can. Health and wellness is a journey to be experienced by the individual. I realize that this too has flow and some people are just not a vibrational match for what we teach at this moment. I also realize that pushing you forward when you are not really ready yet would be like helping a caterpillar out of its cocoon – destructive.

CHAPTER 13

FALLING DOWN AND GETTING UP AGAIN

AS WE HAVE EXPLORED IN THE PREVIOUS CHAPTERS, BEING healthy and having a healthy sense of well-being requires us to take a step back from the average, everyday American lifestyle. There will be people who choose to implement what's been mentioned in previous chapters and others who will just stop before they ever get started. Creating a healthier lifestyle for yourself and your family is a choice. Sometimes, it is a choice you have to continue to make over and over again, throughout the day, week, or year. Having the support of family members is helpful, but not everyone has that luxury.

Transforming your body and health takes time and patience. You don't expect to lose twenty pounds and keep it off by going to the gym once and doing five push-ups one time. In the same way, reading a book about making lifestyle changes for better health and then eating gluten-free for one day, or even one week, isn't going to get you the results you want.

I can flat-out say that I fall off the wagon. I eat Mexican food a little too often, and when I start to feel out of sorts, tired, and sluggish, I have to remind myself to clean up my act again. Watch out for the little extra pieces of chocolate, the tortilla chips, and the over-processed gluten-free products and cheese. I know that I feel better when I don't eat junk and instead stick with more of a plant-based diet with some quality animal proteins. That doesn't mean that I don't enjoy a meal out now and then. It does, however, mean that I've cut way back on eating out. This lifestyle also means that

I plan and prepare meals at home more and avoid drive-through restaurants and chemicals as much as possible. Once I found products and product lines that made those choices easier, I didn't have to think so hard or make as much effort to shift. Then, when I come across a new food, way of exercising, or cleaning product that is an upgrade from what I'm currently doing, I change again.

The holidays are always challenging, as going home to family is like trying to squeeze back in a round hole when I have no doubts that I am square now. I take my own food and often prepare some for the whole family. My family has not shifted to an organic, gluten-free, low-processed, low-added sugar diet, but they have taken on some of the less toxic products I've recommended because they've realized those foods work better for them compared with what they previously ate too. We can't expect everyone in our circle to follow what we do. All we can do is prepare our best and accept that there are going to be some things that aren't our new usual.

A few years ago when I started this journey, I had prepared well for Thanksgiving – I brought gluten free flour, a hormone-free turkey and all the ingredients for gluten free cornbread dressing. Then, when I went to shower, my mom threw regular flour in the roasting bag with the turkey. When I realized what she had done, I stopped further gluten contamination by using chicken broth instead of the broth out of the turkey she would usually use in the dressing to keep it gluten free, and only had turkey for that one meal. When eating leftovers, I only ate ham and chicken and things other than the turkey. This sort of thing happens and you just have to choose the best course of action in the moment. Getting angry or not eating with the family wouldn't be beneficial to anyone. If I had celiac's disease, I just wouldn't have eaten it, but minor exposure to a sensitivity on rare occasion has a lesser impact than continued cheats on a regular basis. As your body heals, you may be able to handle having some of these foods back in your diet.

You are creating a new relationship with your Self. In doing so, and as the newness wears off, it will be easy to slip back into old habits. Additionally, as you begin feeling better, it is easy to just go back to what you did before. This is the perfect way to get back to where you started, or worse. This is why dieting rarely works. Anyone can do something for a short period of time, but when it comes to making choices day-in and day-out, the easy path is the one of least resistance.

People fail at transforming their lives and bodies because they stay surrounded by what has always been there. People go to same grocery stores and have the same patterns of watching TV, playing computer games, drinking alcohol, and eating out. People also have the same friends, who somehow don't seem to be noticing the effects of their toxic diet and lifestyle.

This is why I like to create this lifestyle change as a group project where you have others who have similar struggles, challenges, successes, triumphs, and mishaps going through the changes with you. Trust me, mishaps happen. The other day, I cooked spaghetti for dinner with friends; my one friend and I eat a vegetable version of noodles (zoodles, palm noodles, or spaghetti squash) and her husband eats pasta. As we prepared the noodles, she asked how I knew if they were done, and as old habits die hard, I popped the end of one in my mouth to see if the pasta was tender. It wasn't until about ten seconds later, that I processed that was wheat, although I haven't eaten wheat in four years (at least, that I knew of!) In my case, that one teeny bite made no difference, but for my friends with celiac disease, it could be catastrophic. This is exactly why I don't keep wheat and other allergens in my own home, as it is easy to forget.

Many people never start to clean up their diet and surroundings, even when they have heard of the benefits. It either seems like too much effort or they just don't believe that they can succeed at feeling better. It is much easier to stay stuck and eventually decline enough that you will be given the "magic pill," which isn't all that magic. The majority of people on medications, while their lab numbers may look "normal," don't completely feel better or have instead traded one set of symptoms for a whole new set. I think of this like cleaning a house. I don't love cleaning my house, but I do love waking up to a clean kitchen and walking into a clean bathroom. I love the sense of peace when things are in their proper places instead of strewed and cluttered around. If we never cleaned our houses, or only took out the trash once a month, it would be uncomfortable to live there. It's the same with our bodies.

Personally, this lifestyle becomes an act of self-love and respect. I choose not to eat the things that clog up my body with toxicity or cause inflammation. To support my body, I take supplements for foods that I don't think I will ever choose to eat – like liver – or foods that I know are depleted from the environment. The more I listen to my intuition and honor my own inner guidance, the stronger I get, the less tired I feel, and the more inspired I am to reach out and make a difference in the world.

When you are "in it," (the emotions, lifestyle, mind-set, etc.) it can be hard to see a way out. It may seem like nothing you do makes a difference. Notice that this is the signal, the sign on your roadmap to a healthier life. Shifting to use the tools you've learned and the knowledge you now have will give you the option of choice.

At Be Zen Holistic Wellness Center, we offer individual sessions, coaching, acupuncture, labs, supplements, meal plans, and more in our Allen, Texas, clinic. In addition, we work with individuals virtually throughout the United States. Our group programs are based on the information in this book and include lab work and individualized supplements, with the added experience of working with a group, having live videos, and enjoying recipes, group meditations, clearings, nutrition classes, and more. Many functional medicine clinics do labs and suggest diet and lifestyle changes – some even have group programs – but few have a traditional Chinese medicine foundation and work with the mindset, emotional, and spiritual connections like we do. So, I invite you to join us!

CHAPTER 14

ENLIGHTENMENT – FEELING LIGHTER

YOUR DOCTOR WAS RIGHT; YOUR LABS WERE "NORMAL," AND you are getting older. Hopefully now you understand that "normal" is a setting on your dryer or washing machine and that all bodies are different. Eating right and exercising are important parts of staying healthy, but optimal health for you is going to look different than it does for your husband, wife, neighbor, mom, friends, coworkers, or anyone else.

The biggest thing to remember is that every step you take toward living a healthier lifestyle is a step in the right direction. Even baby steps will get you where you want to go if you are consistently moving forward. It often can feel like a few steps forward and one or two steps back, but when the overall motion is forward, you are on your way to feeling better.

Your higher Self has been gently nudging you (maybe with a two by four) to make changes in your life. So, I have laid out a map for you to do so. Your higher Self and physical body both respond to changes in your energetic, emotional, and mind bodies. Here's a quick recap of what we learned about each body to remind you what we went through.

To eliminate the symptoms of low thyroid as well as most other chronic health problems from a physical body perspective, you need to clean up your diet and surroundings (wood), get more quality sleep (fire), eliminate foods that you have allergies and sensitivities to (earth), have regular bowel movements (metal), and drink more clean water (water).

The energetic body is reflected in your physical symptoms. If you are tired, sluggish, constipated, and cold, your energetic body is not moving as well as it ideally should be. Putting into action the processes mentioned in each chapter will be helpful in getting both the energetic and the physical back up to speed and running optimally.

The mind-body is always a work in progress. Even masters of personal growth and development are always working on themselves and learning new things. It is a process and every time you think you have done the work, some old pattern comes around again. I think of this more like a higher level of the same old stuff or like an upward rising spiral. Each time it comes around, it moves through the cycle in less time and with more clarity. Instead of beating yourself up, consider the pattern an old friend that reminds you of where you came from.

The emotional body is a highly evolved indicator system to tell us where we are struggling to find balance—not the yin-yang, pivotal, teeter-totter balance, but the balancing-a-plate-on-one-finger sort of balance. When we learn to observe our emotions and understand the signals they give us, it gives us the ability to not only heal ourselves but also the ones around us when we give witness to their pain. Suffering is optional when you understand that each emotion leads to an action that puts the next element into play.

Water may bring fear, but the contraction and turning inward allows us to rest and shows us our next best move. Wood brings growth, sometimes through anger to raise our vibration, so that we attract fire, as well as the relationships that support us and bring joy. Earth grounds us in a new way of being and self-expression. Metal may bring grief, but it reminds us to let go when it is time and to not hold on too tightly to it, as nothing is permanent. Change is the one thing we are guaranteed will happen and fear of the unknown can be the opportunity to turn inward and grow, or else the freeze, fight, or flight impulse will keep us stuck.

Enlightenment is not a magical state reserved for those who live in monasteries on mountaintops and do nothing but meditate and focus on mindfulness. It is those baby steps that lighten your load. Any and every act that allows you to feel lighter, more connected, and more at peace with your Self is enlightenment.

What is possible now? That is up to you. What do you want to do? Is it as simple as walking the front yard with the dog today, or is your dream bigger – do you want to climb a mountain or run a marathon? What is something you have always wanted to do but never have? Start seeing it as a possibility for you to create relationships with those who would support you, gather resources, let go of the naysayers and negative mind-talk, and then rest and make it happen. You've got this!

Acknowledgments

I am so grateful for the years that my patients asked, "Is there a book I can read that will tell me about that 'voo doo' that you do?" Their curiosity and willingness to embrace my thoughts and stories encourages me still. Without you, the inspiration, magic, and wisdom of these pages would have never come to be. You inspire me to be and do my best.

Printed in the United States
by Baker & Taylor Publisher Services